In the hierarchical corporate world, [barcode] *slowly corrode the time we have for increasing sense of isolation and co* souls. *This book is an honest, vulnerable and open collection of real-life stories, shared by the brave and collated to create an important sense of community and feels like an important and relevant conversation starter for so many men. Some challenges are personal and at times can seem over-bearing, Philip's book is a reminder that we are not alone and no matter how dark a situation may seem there is a way forward.*

Steve Leeson, Global Head of Talent, Elixirr Consulting

Real people, real stories, and real-life solutions, Men Speak Up *is a much-needed collection of real people sharing how they found themselves struggling with depression, anxiety, addictions, chronic health conditions, and the ever-present day-to-day challenges we all face. The raw vulnerability shared in these narratives is sure to resonate with you and provide you with some guidance to take your next step or maybe your first step to improve your life!*

Mark Meier, MSW, LICSW – Founder, The Face It Foundation, USA

This book breaks the taboo of discussing men's mental health. Fourteen brave men and women speak up about their mental health issues, normalising them and providing strategies they used to cope. This book shows we are not individuals grappling with insurmountable problems but a community that needs to find better ways of communicating and sharing our lived experiences so we can all cope a little bit better with life.

Professor Mark Maslin FRGS, FRSA – Professor of Earth System Science at UCL

MEN
SPEAK UP

Journeys Through
Mental Health

PHILIP BRISCOE

Paperback ISBN: 978-1-0685247-0-7

eBook ISBN: 978-1-0685247-1-4

Cover and interior design: Andy Meaden, meadencreative.com

DISCLAIMER

Men Speak Up: Journeys Through Mental Health is based on interviews with people who have experienced a range of mental health challenges.

These experiences include discussions of depression, anxiety, suicide, trauma, substance abuse, and other sensitive topics. Some readers may find these accounts distressing or triggering.

This book is not intended to be a substitute for professional medical advice, diagnosis, or treatment. These are personal stories, reflecting individual experiences: they should not be considered a form of therapy, coaching, or medical guidance.

If you or someone you know is facing mental health concerns, it is crucial to seek help from a qualified professional, such as a doctor, general practitioner, psychiatrist, or licensed therapist. This book does not provide any medical advice, treatment strategies, or therapeutic guidance.

Always consult with a healthcare provider before making any decisions about your mental health or well-being.

To the people who have spoken up,
and to those who are still finding the
strength to do so – this book is for you.

CONTENTS

ACKNOWLEDGEMENTS

This book is a direct result of the *Mid-Life Men* podcast, which I began in early 2023 with the aim of helping men talk more openly about their mental health. Over the past couple of years, I've been privileged to speak to so many individuals and I want to thank each and every one for trusting me with their stories and allowing me to share them with the world in the hope of helping others.

The 14 stories featured in this book are drawn from those podcast episodes, and it was a tough decision to select which ones to include. Please know that every guest, whether featured here or not, has contributed immensely to this important conversation, and I am deeply grateful to all of you.

To the people featured in the book, your honesty and willingness to show vulnerability is a testament to the strength it takes to talk about mental health, and I am humbled and sincerely thankful.

To everyone who has encouraged and supported me along this journey, from the podcast's beginnings to the creation of this book, I am truly thankful. Your belief in the importance of this work has kept me going, especially during the tougher moments.

To my family, I cannot thank you enough. You have been my constant support, giving me the space and time I needed, even when it meant ridiculously early morning sessions and long hours spent focused on this project. A huge thank you to my wife, Elspeth, for your patience and understanding and for taking the dogs out when they started to get rowdy to give me a bit of peace and quiet.

Finally, a special thanks to Robert, my copyeditor, whose keen attention to detail – and thoughtful suggestions – helped me shape this book into its best form.

This journey has been one of shared voices and collective strength. Thank you all for being part of it.

FOREWORD

Philip Briscoe is to be congratulated on *Men Speak Up*. He has brought together stories from a range of men discussing their varied struggles with mental health. Their narratives capture the reality of recovery, which involves learning to live well – whether that means with or beyond mental health issues.

Stories told about mental health recovery can sometimes be idealised, starting with psychological distress arising from emotional problems or early adverse experiences, and then describing an ever-improving trajectory towards well-being through health behaviours, relationships and lifestyle choices. This 'master narrative' of illness moving inexorably to health is neat and tidy, but doesn't capture the messy reality of most people's lives. What is particularly powerful about this book is how the narrators bravely confront the causes, experiences and responses to mental health problems. The stories locate mental health issues within the broader identity of being a man. Topics covered include the helpful and harmful aspects of alcohol, careers, crime, drugs (prescribed and recreational), ego, exercise, gambling, health problems, laziness, music, mutual support, parenting, porn, resilience, sexual performance, sport, suicide, therapy, violence and trauma, weakness and vulnerability. These important aspects of being are discussed bravely, honestly and authentically.

Why do stories matter? My research group (Recovery Research Team, University of Nottingham) has focused for many years on the impact of 'recovery narratives'. In our Narrative Experiences Online (NEON) study described at researchintorecovery.com/neon, we define a recovery narrative as:

a. a first-person lived experience account, i.e. the person tells their own story

b. describing elements of both adversity/struggle and of strength/success/survival, although the positive aspects may be a very small part to a very large part of the story

c. related at least in part to mental health problems, i.e. is about recovery but might relate to escape (e.g. from damaging services, from a negative sense of self), enlightenment (e.g. making new sense of experiences, survivor mission) or endurance (e.g. 'I'm still here', 'I have survived')

d. one that refers to events or actions over a period of time (i.e. is a story).

Based on this definition, *all* of the stories in this book are recovery narratives.

In our research we developed an empirical model of how recovery narratives can impact on people reading them. The ability to connect to the narrator and the narrative content emerges as a key source of impact. This connection leads to comparison, learning and empathy, all of which can benefit the person reading the story. The great strength of this book is the focus on a particular type of narrator (men) and the diversity of narrative content making meaningful connection more possible. These authentic and multifaceted stories provide a rich resource to benefit other people of all genders who are living with mental health issues and who may be earlier in their recovery journey. Learning how people come through hardship to a better life, comparing and empathising with stories, and sometimes just knowing you're not alone, can all be sources of hope and meaning in life.

I hope that this book will be widely read, both by men who find themselves on their own mental health recovery journey, and by those around them – friends, family, colleagues – who might recommend it to someone who is struggling. It eloquently addresses the silence that can occur in relation to men's mental health, and contains many nuggets of wisdom emerging from this lived experience. I fully recommend it.

Mike Slade
Professor of Mental Health Recovery and Social Inclusion
University of Nottingham
October 2024

PREFACE

Although male mental health awareness is increasing, issues like depression, anxiety, and addiction often remain hidden. The consequences of this are alarming: rising rates of male suicide, drug and alcohol abuse, and work-related stress.

Cultural norms and stigmas continue to hold back conversations about mental health, preventing men from seeking the support they need. Many men still feel embarrassed, fearful of being judged, or ill-equipped to share their struggles with even those closest to them.

I know from personal experience that maintaining good mental health is a delicate balance – and I know how quickly things can change. No one is immune and most of us have experienced, or will experience, struggles at some point in our lives. Looking around, I felt that there was a lack of resources focused on supporting men and I wanted to do something to help fill the void.

In early 2023, I had the idea to start a story-based podcast, *Mid-Life Men*, talking to men about their mental health challenges. This book is the next iteration of the podcast. It is an edited collection of 14 stories, each one honest and often raw, told by the men (and two women) who have lived them. Whatever their age, nationality or hardship, these are all remarkable people. Their openness is the real strength behind this collection; they are unafraid of appearing vulnerable and broken. It is easy to use words like 'brave' or 'courageous', but every narrator is unequivocal in their desire to share their experiences to benefit others. There is such immense power in hearing others tell their stories, especially when they resonate with your own.

What I aim to demonstrate, in sharing these first-hand accounts, is that talking about mental health isn't a sign of weakness – *it's a sign of strength.*

The book is for everyone: the men who are struggling, feeling isolated or lost; the loved ones who don't know how to help; and even those who may not yet realise they need some support. Each chapter provides a reminder that you are not alone, and that there can be a path forward to something better. And if any of these stories helps just one person realise they can speak up, or maybe even saves a life, then the book has done its job.

Philip Briscoe

PAUL H
DON'T HIDE YOUR DEPRESSION: IT CAN SAVE YOUR LIFE

'There was a friend of mine who was going through something similar, and we would meet up and we would talk about suicidal thoughts and in funny situations – for example, when we're stood in a cake shop, looking at a Bakewell tart, thinking: "Should we just carry on talking about suicide while we're in here and the different ways you can do it?" It was just really nice to talk to somebody who got it, you know.'

It's hard to pinpoint when it actually properly started. I'd had several years where I'd been feeling a bit like things were not quite right, a bit uncertain. I'd been working at a particular company for 15 years. I'd effectively gone from school, from A-levels, into accountancy training, and felt like this was the right path. This was the answer. I didn't want to go to university, because I was a bit shy at that point and it didn't appeal to me. I was good with numbers and maths at school and then an opportunity came up to become a trainee accountant. So, I did it.

I started to become more successful, and I found myself leading the finances for a construction company. It was exciting for a period, but I think, over the last several years, it just felt like I was living a bit of a lie. I was living a life I didn't really want to, and I thought: 'Is this normal? Is this what we're supposed to do?' And I assumed it was. I think it all stems from when I was younger. Being brought up, we were reasonably well off, so I thought it was the case that you're supposed to put on a show, and it is supposed to be all about status and chasing material wealth, and now I was starting to slowly realise that wasn't the answer for me.

A big part of it was I wasn't getting any fulfilment at work, because what you find with accounts is that, once you've got things working well, it kind of looks after itself and comes to a point where it's all running okay. Generally, people in business often don't value accounts in the finance team that much and it felt like I was just a cog in the wheel.

Even though businesses talk about looking after the staff and fulfilment and other things, ultimately the driver is that it's a capitalist world and it's about profits, and it's also people's own wealth, ego, and status, and I would sit in board meetings and just be thinking: 'What am I doing?' These people are bothered about bonuses, they're bothered about status, then they talk about softer skills, but how much do they genuinely buy into that?

I think a big part of what this mid-life challenge becomes is that a lot of people realise: 'Oh, look, I've ended up living a life I don't really want to live', and this is what happened to me. I wasn't doing what I wanted to do.

If I had my chance again, and somebody had talked to me about what I truly wanted to do and what I enjoyed doing (which is an exercise I've done recently), it would have steered me in a different direction. Definitely.

I had the chance to take voluntary redundancy. I thought that I needed to move on anyway and this was an opportunity for me to do so, especially as I was having doubts about my career and its direction.

$$\star\,\star\,\star$$

There were elements of a bit of anger management when I was younger, but just really questioning things. I was getting frustrated quite easily. I tend to have a short fuse anyway, and there were more instances of anger, of not being content, and a lot of questioning my own value, and the value I brought to work and to the world, essentially, on a bigger scale. It manifested as a cloud and was getting heavier and bigger over time, and that was magnified when there were the added pressures of a change of job. I hid it. I was not at that point showing my true self to people.

Taking voluntary redundancy was definitely a big trigger for a higher level of depression and a realisation that I was hunting for something else.

I went into a couple of short-term jobs, but they didn't feel right and there were mornings when I just didn't want to go to work. I would feel very emotional. So that cloud was always there in the morning, as soon as I woke up. During the day, it was always there and I wanted to escape, but I was like: 'How do I escape from this?'

And quite quickly, I was regularly having suicidal thoughts, especially in the bad moments when perhaps I'd overreacted, or had a drink. It just seemed the easiest way out and it became quite normal for me to have these thoughts, but I wouldn't share them with people.

I felt sad and very lonely, even in my own house. I've got two kids and a wife, but I would often hide away from them. I was lonely because people didn't understand. I didn't have somebody to talk to who understood, and obviously you can't put it on your kids, and I couldn't burden my wife with it.

There were often times I would say to myself: 'I'm on my own.' Even my friends, some of whom were going through similar things, would want to give me advice but I just wanted to be heard.

The thing about the suicidal thoughts is, because I had a family, I didn't feel that that it was something I could do; it wasn't a realistic escape. I also didn't know what it entailed, and

I didn't want the pain of it. There were a couple of instances where I was out and about, and I was on this bridge and there was a sign on the bridge advertising the Samaritans.

I looked over the bridge and I just thought: 'Could I jump off this bridge?' And at the time I didn't think I could, out of fear. It made me understand that some people must get to a really bad place where fear doesn't become a factor that stops them. Thankfully, I had factors like my family. So, instead I started to look for easier ways out.

There was one time, when I was having a bad time, I hadn't been running regularly for a long time and I decided I was just going to go for a run – and I was going to run until my heart stopped. I wanted to find a way out that would mean my family would be alright. I had health insurance. I would have just died while out running, and it wouldn't be something I had to do to myself. So, I went out and just kept running, and running, and running in the hope that my body would give up.

So, there were moments like that when you just feel really sad, and you just don't know the way out. I didn't want to live this life any more, and it felt like there was no easy answer or quick fix.

I think a tipping point for me was when I was regularly hiding from my family, I wanted to sleep more, and I was having regular suicidal thoughts. That was ultimately when I felt like I needed to do something different. It makes me emotional just recalling these moments.

You just want to escape somehow. For me, escape meant I wanted to go out in nature. I wanted to go to a hut in the middle of nowhere and escape the real world. Whatever way it was defined, it was ultimately about escaping this life, this cloud, this feeling.

* * *

Being somebody who always questions a lot and needs answers, I was investing a lot of time in reading and trying to find other ways of finding joy, but nothing was clicking. There were certain books that I quite liked, including Eckhart Tolle's books: *A New Earth* and *The Power of Now*. I was trying to explore mindfulness and being in the moment and it resonated with me, this book about a new earth, egos, and getting out of the corporate world. All of a sudden, I was starting to find that maybe there's a different way to find joy. There's a different way to be happy and to live your life that doesn't revolve around chasing a goal. You can actually try and live now, and I had been struggling with that. It made sense to me, but it's something you really need to practise.

Over the years, I've dropped in and out and seen different types of counsellors, and therapists, just to understand a bit more about me and find answers. I think what I'm finding out now with a therapist is that I'm somebody who wants answers and knowledge. So, there was always an element of exploring why I felt like I did and what I wanted, but I never quite understood why.

I saw a cognitive behavioural therapy counsellor, virtually, for a short period of time, which was okay to a degree, but I didn't feel it quite worked for me.

Then I came across psychotherapy and I felt like that was what I needed: someone to really analyse what was going on. I found a psychotherapist and life coach, and fortunately she was local to me.

On reflection, this was the best thing I did: finding a good-quality therapist and working with her to explore the life-coaching aspects, the wellness coaching, and exploring who I am and what I want to do. There was a lot about me learning what my passions were, the stuff that I should have done when I was younger. We went through steps to explore my personality type, what I enjoy, what I get lost in, but one of the biggest things is that it provides a safe space where you can go and talk to somebody and it's just about you.

If you find a good therapist that you connect with, that's great, you know, where you can just talk, talk, and talk, but the biggest thing she's done is give me permission. Permission to do a variety of things, but ultimately permission to prioritise me and live my life. That's something that has made a massive difference. As a husband and dad, often I feel I need to do this or that. She said: 'For one, your kids are happy that you're just there; you don't have to do everything, you know?' That was a bit of a revelation for me. I'm able to now start prioritising myself. That was very much the beginning of working towards a road to recovery.

I think therapy is comparable to anything where it's easier to have a specialist helping you. It's very hard to fix yourself reading books, because you need the massive power you get from having a therapist and a professional, and they'll narrow down to the important things. But one thing that a therapist can tell you is that you don't need to find the answers to everything.

Every time I go to a session, at the end of it I've got this new-found clarity and it's more an emotional thing. I think people massively benefit from having somebody there who's on their side. You'll have people close to you who care for you, friends who care for you, but they're living with their own problems, their own lives, and they're not trained. But to have somebody for an hour or whatever who is absolutely focused on helping you – that's invaluable.

Going to these therapy sessions is somebody saying: 'You don't have to do that, you don't have to do this, you can give yourself a break.' And when you hear it from other people, it's more powerful because we're a lot nicer to other people than we are to ourselves. I think there's definitely value in working with somebody else.

* * *

I think there are a few things that make a big difference. Try and put yourself out there authentically – that's what I did in my post on LinkedIn. It was my way of putting myself out there. I was fearful about it, and I was very honest about what I'd been going through. And the response I got from people, including directors and CEOs, was that they're going through the same thing. I think they're just not comfortable with putting themselves out there.

Talk authentically about what you're feeling. Be honest, be vulnerable. I realise now that LinkedIn is a community of human beings who are vulnerable. I look at all these successful people and they've all got problems – so be vulnerable.

Explore a psychotherapist or a wellness life coach, because they make a massive difference. You can do it virtually. You can do it face to face. Search on the internet for different people. They can have one of the biggest impacts by providingthat safe space that allows you to be you, and to prioritise yourself.

If you feel like you are living a life that's not you, there is to a degree a certain switch where you can just go: 'I'm not going to live that lie any more.' And I know there are different levels of lies that people are faced with – because of cultural norms or whatever – but, as much as you can, live authentically; it makes a massive difference.

The thing about me reading Eckhart Tolle books about the ego is that my ego gets me into a lot of problems. It gets me angry. It gets me kicking off or upset about what people think. So, explore things where you could take the ego out of it. Just try and be you, and it's alright. Think: 'I'm going to take my ego out and I'm going to put myself out there.'

* * *

I started taking antidepressants maybe four or five months ago. I'd avoided it up until that point, just because I didn't want to be dependent on them and I wanted to try and tackle it in a more natural way, but there was an instance where I smashed a cup in the living room and I was like: 'I can't be feeling like this all the time.' So, I started taking a low dose of them and, at first, I didn't really tell people – but then I started openly admitting it. And again, it was just a weight off my shoulders. It doesn't matter. There are a lot of people on these tablets, but it's just one tool that you can use to help, and my therapist was saying it can help, but you just don't want to be too dependent on it.

I think that if I'd had somebody explaining to me what life can be about rather than it being about chasing that great career, with the answer at the end of the rainbow when you get to a certain financial stability and wealth, I think I would have had a much more satisfying life up until now.

The corporate world now works well for me because I've adapted it in a way that's more satisfying, more human, and I'm helping people using softer skills rather than it just being a big PLC that you can get lost in. For me, there's a definite adaption and learning, which is why working with small and medium-sized companies just feels so much more satisfying. These are family-run businesses, and their lives are massively dependent on the success of their businesses. So, a human-to-human interaction is a lot more authentic.

I'm adding on wellness coaching and personal training [PT] because I very much have an interest in that, and I'm focused on mid-lifers. I think if somebody had managed to unlock the realisation that I want to help people in the mental health space, I think I would have felt so much more alive for so much longer. And I think that's the difference I felt, throughout my career, where it just didn't feel right.

I do think there's an education piece about the capitalist world and not being too ego-driven, which impacts mental health generally in society. We're all brought up and trained at school. My daughter's school is seen as a bit of a business school, and they're encouraged to wear suits when they get into sixth form, and I just think: 'Is that the only way?'

I think it's more about creating community and helping each other. For example, I used to be a massive England fan and a Formula One fan. I'd get so caught up in it, whereas now I'm trying to embrace the fact that, whether they win or lose, it doesn't matter. I've realised the joy you can get from enjoying other people's success and it's a natural joy. So, I think if there'd been somebody at school who taught me about these natural ways that you can get joy, enjoying now and not chasing something at the end, I think I would have been in a much better place. And I think a lot of mid-lifers would be.

I think we're sold a bit of a lie when we're younger and we end up following something on the trust that, well, 'I've been to school, I've got all these qualifications, and so I'm set up for life.' I think we're setting up a lot of people to hit mid-life and realise it is not true; but society, and the way that we are a capitalist world, is just geared up to this.

So ultimately, for me now, I want to use my qualifications and I want to build on the PT and wellness to help mid-lifers, because I have felt the pain that they will be going through. But I want to at some point try and impact a younger generation too. Get a message out that there is another way.

There are a lot of people in this position, who are having career changes late on. It's just another sign that we don't quite get it right sometimes. There are different ways. Definitely.

I think the thing is, from my experience, people just want to be heard; that's the biggest thing. As much as you can, be there to hear them, to listen to them. It's not about trying to fix them, because I would have friends giving me advice, and there were times when I didn't want advice. The main element was that feeling of being on your own.

There was a friend of mine who was going through something similar, and we would meet up and we would talk about suicidal thoughts and in funny situations – for example, when we're stood in a cake shop, looking at a Bakewell tart, thinking: 'Should we just carry on talking about suicide while we're in here and the different ways you can do it?' It was just really nice to talk to somebody who got it, you know, whereas if you mention it to your partner or whatever, it's a big word.

At the end of the day, there'll always be ups and downs. The last day or so I've had a bit of a down. At the moment I'm going through training, doing a PT body transformation, trying to get stronger and healthier for me, and it has massively helped doing some coaching and wellness. And these are all things that I focused on in my new purpose; it's definitely driving me and it's releasing me from the cloud, and I feel like I'm working towards an answer, but there are days when I'm suddenly reminded of that cloud, that feeling, and that's okay.

I'm learning to allow myself to experience that and, as it goes up and down, just to ride it out. There'll be days when you'll feel like it's not that bad. And then there'll be days where you'll really struggle. Whatever the feeling, it's just good to talk.

I think, overall, just try and live your life authentically, be true to yourself, and definitely explore seeing a psychotherapist – that would be my advice.

If you are not happy and it doesn't feel right, it may not be an instant fix, but you need to take ownership, have faith in the process, and try not to worry about where you will get to. You will find your superpower and the answer at the end.

JAMES
BETTING IT ALL: HOW GAMBLING ALMOST TOOK MY LIFE

'A rational-thinking person would not forge their bank statement and try and get money from a payday loan company with a thousand per cent interest. It was not a rational thought, and that's what gambling addiction does to you.'

So first and foremost, I am in recovery from a 12-year gambling addiction, and that has played a big part in the job that I have now, which is leading a campaign to get gambling advertising out of football. I'm also proud to represent Gambling with Lives [https://www.gamblingwithlives.org], which is a charity set up by bereaved families who had lost loved ones to gambling-related suicide, and my role is to oversee our education programme for young people.

I'm 34 years old, originally from Norfolk and life is good at the moment.

My exposure to gambling started for me as a child. I'm from a town in Norfolk where there wasn't a lot to do. The only place to gamble was a very small, hidden, windowless, dingy bookie that, as a kid, I remember I was quite scared of. I used to think: 'That's not a place I ever want to go.' Around the age of 16 or 17, in 2007, everything changed with gambling in this country, and all of a sudden we all had access to a casino in our pocket with online gambling.

The small bookie I just described changed into a bright, visible, accessible place in our high street – a huge global brand that took up the space of about three shops and had five or six machines in there, with freebie offers outside.

At the same time that was happening, advertising and sponsorship of gambling became widespread and especially so in the sport that I had loved all my life: football.

At that point in my life, every time I watched football, I felt I was encouraged to gamble. And at 16, one day on our lunch break from sixth form, with the bookie only a two-minute walk, me and my mates went in.

We knew the manager. He didn't ask any questions, didn't check our ages, and I put on a £5 football bet. At 16. That was the start of a 12-year addiction.

* * *

What I would like to do at this point is to challenge some perceptions of gambling and gambling addiction.

I had a great upbringing. I had an amazing family. I had a good life. I was motivated and doing well at school. I was off to university. I had a hundred things on my wall, like literally a hundred things written down that I wanted to achieve before I was 30. I had my whole life ahead of me, and I feel strongly that gambling found me, at that ripe and susceptible age of 16.

To challenge another perception: I don't feel like I have an addictive personality. That's something that you may hear quite a lot. I've never been addicted to anything else. I've never had any other problems in my life. Yes, I've had things go wrong like everybody does, but there's been no other main thing that's caused so much harm to me as gambling did. I just had a random contact with an addictive product at an age where my brain wasn't fully developed, and that's what created 12 years of just horrible, awful, devastating addiction.

There were a number of people in that town that I've now come to learn had addiction problems too. I think as well, being from that small town with not a lot to do, you can't escape the fact that we probably used gambling as a bit of escapism because there was nothing much more to do. Obviously, it wasn't just my town; millions of people have been harmed by the gambling industry.

* * *

What caused the addiction? Good question. I didn't have a big first win, but it's so common in stories of gambling addiction that a young person, or anyone who gambles, in the early stages of their gambling journey experiences a big first win.

And what happens in your brain is an explosion of dopamine. You can't believe that you've been able to win this money, and so then the brain is constantly trying to replicate this feeling, and so you try and use more money to recreate that same feeling. I now work with young people, and I say to them that actually if you do get a big first win you may think you are quite lucky, but I would say, actually, you are quite unlucky because your brain will now genuinely try and get that feeling back again and again and again.

The addiction really happened for me because, though I started with football betting, when I went to place bets in the bookies there were also highly addictive, fast-paced roulette machines that used to be £100 a spin maximum.

Now, thanks to a high-profile campaign and government action, the maximum bet has been reduced to £2. But, as a child, I was playing them, and they have addiction rates of somewhere between 30 per cent and 40 per cent. So, these genuinely harmful products were available on our high streets, promoted everywhere we looked, and that's when I really, really felt addicted. When I started going into the bookies, I would go by myself, when my friends weren't there, and not tell people where I was going. I used to lie about my gambling. I used to hide behind the machines if my mum was walking past doing her shopping, because I was ashamed. Even at that age, I was ashamed that I couldn't go a day without gambling.

Then when I had access to online gambling, well, that was a complete disaster because I didn't need to go into the bookies, and I didn't need to worry about hiding any more. I didn't need to worry about lying about where I'd been because I could just do it in bed. I could do it on the sofa, I could do it during lessons. I was a football coach, and I was gambling online whilst I was coaching kids playing football. That's how bad it got. And I was only 18 years old.

And when I went to university, I had access to what I thought at the time was free money – student loans and grants – and free time, and I now know both of those things are not free.

And that was it. I was spending all of that time and money on gambling sites. I ended up having accounts with about a hundred different betting sites and not at any point did a gambling company ask me if I could afford to lose the money I was losing, or if I was okay. Instead, what they did was give me free bets, free spins, and they put me on a VIP scheme, which is where they rewarded me for losing a lot of money by giving me free tickets to Premier League matches, or a day at the horse racing. And this was when I was on minimum wage. Didn't have a pot to piss in.

And I wasn't a VIP by any stretch of the imagination, and they were essentially grooming my illness, and I now look back and think that was deeply irresponsible.

* * *

I recently got my data back from an online gambling company. You can ask for it back through a freedom of information request. And it's not the money that I look at and regret, but I look at the times and the dates that I was gambling and there were days where I would start gambling at 2 a.m. and that's not an exaggeration. I was setting my alarm to bet on football all around the world, or tennis all around the world.

And then just going throughout the day, betting on different sports, playing online slots, online roulette, blackjack, poker, it became completely all-consuming. The idea of watching sports without a bet on would make me shiver, and it became the only thing that I wanted to do. And it is that all-consuming nature: the first thing that I thought about when I woke up and the last thing that I thought about before I went to bed. And I remember thinking: 'This is my life. This is all I'm here to do. I will never have a life that isn't like this.' I couldn't imagine a life without gambling.

Of course, this has such an impact because if you are focused on gambling so much, everything else is a complete distraction or a barrier between you and your addiction.

I'm not going to say that there is no fun caused by gambling. If people didn't take some form of pleasure from it, they wouldn't do it. Actually, I think that the fun and pleasure is a chemical reaction. It's when you win. It's not about winning the money. It's about that feeling of 'Wow, I've got all of these things' and it's made even more so by the bright lights and the noises and just the overwhelming presence of these products.

And eventually what happens is that the fun runs out and I got to a point where I preferred to lose than win, because the idea of winning meant that I had to carry on doing this thing that I knew was destroying my life. If I lost, I knew that I'd lost all my money and I couldn't go back to it.

The money I was using to gamble was rarely mine. It was money I was getting through payday loans. I had 20 payday loans at one point. I was forging my bank statement using a simple graphics editing software tool and sending it to a payday loan company to pretend that I was earning more money than I was. They would give me the money. Within minutes, my bank would accept the money, and then I'd deposit that money straight onto a gambling site without any question from any party involved at all. So, of course, I take responsibility for my recovery, but in that process, a payday loan company, a bank, and a gambling site accepted money that was basically fraudulent without any question at all. That's not acceptable.

* * *

My addiction started making me do things that I never thought I'd do. It turned a perfectly normal, bright, happy, motivated young lad into a very pessimistic, nihilistic, miserable, depressed, anxious, lying wreck of a man.

I did things that I'm not proud of and that I still have the shame and guilt about. A rational-thinking person would not forge their bank statement and try and get money from a payday loan company with a thousand per cent interest. It was not a rational thought, and that's what gambling addiction does to you.

It changes you; it changes the way you think and feel and behave, and that's really hard to overcome. There were times when I honestly thought that I was in control, but the reality was that I was never in control from the minute I placed that first bet.

There were a couple of occasions where my friends sat me down on the sofa – I can still picture it now – and said 'James, you're a gambling addict.' And my response was 'No, I'm not', because that sense of denial meant that I could carry on feeding my addiction. That's what my brain and my addicted brain wanted to do. So, accepting that I was addicted would've meant inevitably getting to that moment where I had to stop, and I wasn't in a place to do that.

There were a lot of moments throughout my addiction where I asked myself: 'How did I get here? Why did nobody warn me? I can't keep doing this.' I cried myself to sleep a lot. I remember sleeping in a train station because I didn't have any money to stay anywhere for a couple of nights. And at that moment it was a real 'Wow, how have I got to this place? I'm not stupid. I feel like I have control over every part of my life other than this addiction.'

But there was one moment, which happens to be the last moment I ever gambled, which was when the bailiffs were coming round to collect against a debt. I felt trapped. I felt hopeless, and I got paid for some work I was doing, and my addicted brain said to me the way of paying that debt was to gamble, to win it.

And you can guess where this story is going. I lost all of that money within minutes of playing roulette in the bookies and that was it. It felt like a bit of an out-of-body experience. I stumbled home to this basement that I was living in at the time.

And that was it. I didn't know if I wanted to die, but I knew that I didn't want to live like this any more. And for three days I was in a complete pit of misery. I didn't eat – I just sat in my bed upright, crying. I didn't turn my phone on because I didn't want anyone to know where I was or talk to me.

But then, something did happen. I opened my laptop, and I was so addicted to gambling that although I didn't have the money to gamble, I was watching people play roulette on YouTube. And as I was doing that, a documentary popped up about an Irish postman called Tony O'Reilly, who was a gambling addict and came out the other side.

And it was the first time I realised that I'm not the only gambling addict in the world and that it was possible to have a life after this. And that was it. That was the last time I ever gambled and that was six years ago.

The first thing I did was to ring my mum and I told her about how gambling was making me feel. Not just the impact on my money, but this was the first time I said, look, this has changed who I am. I'm depressed. I've been crying for three days in this pit, and that was a massive weight off my shoulders actually talking to people.

I know it's cliché, but that's what saved me. And then I had the same conversation with my best mates, the same conversations with my employers, the same conversation with other members of my family. And that really did save me because it allowed me to tell people what I was feeling and that was a layer of accountability.

After I'd done that, I couldn't go back. I put in place Gamban and Gamstop [gambling-specific blocking software] to ban and block myself from online gambling. I also gave control of my bank account to my mum. That was absolutely crucial. Even if I wanted to gamble, I couldn't.

But actually, there wasn't a great urge or temptation; something genuinely clicked. It was a really big moment for me when I said, 'This is it. I'm not going to do this any more.'

* * *

I was in a hundred thousand pounds' worth of debt. I owed all of those loan companies money; incidentally, or maybe ironically, most of them have now gone bust, which doesn't surprise me because it is not a safe and sustainable type of company. I'm still in debt now and I still have to live with the consequences of that. I can't get a mobile phone contract because my credit score is so bad.

I wish people realised the long-term impact when they see adverts for gambling, because people don't. And this is six years later. I still have the scars, not just financially. I still have the scars mentally. Like my brain doesn't work the same way it did before I found gambling. It's scarred in a way that it doesn't take the same pleasure from normal things. It is used to extreme highs and extreme lows and everyday pleasures, everyday things that should be normal for people, I struggle with, and that's the thing that I regret the most.

At the time, the treatment support for gambling addiction in this country was not great for me. I'm pleased to say that's now improved. There are now specialist NHS addiction clinics across the UK, but I had to just replace gambling with meaningful activities. I moved and went to stay on a friend's sofa in Manchester. And just being away from where I had lived when I was gambling felt like a fresh start – a new me. It really helped.

But recovery isn't easy. It's a bumpy old road. One of the things that I really couldn't do was watch football for months, because every time I watched it I'd see an advert for the thing that I was trying everything in my power not to do.

There was a real key moment when my granddad wasn't very well, and I was caring for him. I was there and he used to get the *Daily Mail* every day. Not a paper I'd buy, but I was reading the *Daily Mail* and there was a story about Jack Ritchie and other people who had sadly taken their own lives because of their gambling addiction, and the stories were being told by their families.

And I was paralysed in my seat reading this because I thought, wow, how close I came to that. But I was also paralysed by the bravery of the families to speak out about gambling addiction and suicide. This was the start of this new chapter for me, and I for the first time began to realise the role of the gambling industry in my addiction.

At the time, I thought I was completely to blame. I thought this was all entirely my fault. I thought I was the one that was placing the bets. I was the one that didn't stop. I was the one that was addicted for 12 years. And actually, they were saying that, partly, the reason this happens is because we have addictive products and because £1.5 billion a year is spent on advertising and marketing in the industry, encouraging us all to gamble all the time.

The responsible gambling narrative, such as slogans like 'When the fun stops, stop', tells people it's all up to you. And that's why I felt the shame, the guilt, and the stigma. And from that moment, I wanted to do something about it, and I wanted to do something for charity, which has been extremely beneficial to my recovery.

***

I have a history of doing bizarre charity things and I had the idea of walking to football clubs that had gambling sponsors on the front of their shirts. At the time this was relevant to 30 clubs in the top two divisions. I decided to walk to eight clubs in three days, 124 miles, and it turned into what is now 'The Big Step' [https://www.the-bigstep.com], a campaign to end all gambling advertising and sponsorship in football, led by people harmed by gambling. We did it to raise money and awareness for the charity Gambling with Lives, it was the first thing we did together, and they were extremely supportive from that moment. It has been a great relationship. They've supported me ever since and, in 2020, I am very proud that they employed me to not just lead this campaign, but also lead an education programme for young people.

Gambling with Lives is a charity that was set up by families bereaved by gambling-related suicide, and at our core we are there to support bereaved families, and sadly we are seeing more, with over 400 suicides a year. Every week, every month, we hear of another life lost, and the family left behind, devastated, but wanting to know what they can do and how we can help.

We have a family support team and a therapist to do exactly that. But beyond that, we campaign vigorously for change. The current gambling laws in this country were written in 2005 before the first smartphone was invented. They are completely unfit and have led, in our opinion, to a lot of addiction, a lot of harm, and deaths too, and we campaign strongly to the government for change.

The reason we have an education programme is that nobody warned me about what could happen. And nobody warned the families that they could potentially lose their children because of gambling. So, we go into schools to talk about the role of the products, the practices, the industry, and the environment, and give young people as much information as possible because even that is a raindrop in an ocean of gambling normalisation. We've been piloting that over the last year and now we're delivering the programme across schools, mainly in Northern Ireland and in Greater Manchester. It's going really well, and we hope to expand and scale.

I'd like to think that we've been quite pivotal in the changes taking place across the gambling industry, especially related to advertising in football, and that's mainly I think because we are the voices of lived experience and it's put a face to this all. We've been supported by academics and by parliamentarians and others, but we've been chipping away at this for the last four years and we turned The Big Step into a full-time campaign to end gambling advertising and sponsorship in football. We never thought this would happen overnight, because we're not naïve, but do see the small steps along the journey. During that time, we've seen the Advertising Standards Authority put a rule in to say that footballers can no longer appear in TV advertisements for gambling, which is quite a big deal, and the Premier League has voluntarily agreed to phase out gambling sponsorship on the front of their shirts. This is a significant acceptance of the harm caused by gambling advertising, but on its own it is incoherent because there are 700 gambling adverts every 90-minute match, so we need to encompass all forms of gambling advertising in football at every level, and in every country.

* * *

The first thing I would say to anyone who feels that they are addicted to gambling is please don't think that whatever harm has happened is all your fault. I would also say: don't think that gambling is the answer to any of the problems that you have. I used to think that the way of getting out of trouble was by gambling more, but it just causes more trouble, and there is no nice, glorious jackpot waiting for you. The industry makes £14 billion a year. It makes the vast majority of its profits from those of us who are addicted or at risk of being so, and 99 per cent of customers lose.

The other 1 per cent either get their account restricted or banned. I'm sorry to say this, but you can't win, and I think I needed to hear that quite early into my addiction. Just think about the things that you can do with a life free from gambling. Football is better without a bet on, I promise you that. Speak to people. Block and ban yourself from gambling websites. And if you're worried about a loved one, look at GamFam [https://gamfam.org.uk], a charity which supports families affected by gambling harm.

Finally, if you do ever come across a family or someone you know who has been bereaved by gambling-related suicide, please do pass them on to the Gambling with Lives charity, because we are there to help them.

JONATHAN
FINDING HUMOUR THROUGH THE DARKNESS: SURVIVING A HEART TRANSPLANT

'But it's you – this is happening to you; your depression is happening to you; your moments of like, "I'm going to commit suicide" are happening to you. No one else. But you have to pause and then take a deep breath and then, you know, tomorrow will be better. You have to have some optimism.'

It was just an ordinary morning. I was taking a shower at 7 a.m. as usual. I remember looking at the shower bottle labels and couldn't read them; it was literally gibberish and could have been written in Greek for all I knew. I managed to get out of the shower, and sit on the toilet – pretty dramatic but, you know, not very glamorous. I couldn't yell, I couldn't scream, I couldn't do anything. Ultimately, my son saw me, and he showed up like: 'What are you doing?' My son and my wife had no idea what was wrong with me, but they called the paramedics, and it wasn't until they arrived that anyone realised I was having a stroke. This was in 2007 and my life in that instant had changed.

So, I had two strokes – massive strokes, by the way – and heart failure. I suffered brain damage – about 15 per cent – and I had aphasia. Aphasia is the inability to speak, and I had to go through speech therapy. I couldn't speak. It took me years to be able to speak again and I still stumble over words; I can't get them out because the connections in my brain were really messed up and are not quite there forever. Also, there is sometimes a disconnect between what I'm thinking I'm saying and what I'm actually saying.

I lost my business. I was producing movies. I came back from a film festival in Utah, and it had been successful. We had sold our movie at the highest sale point. Everything was really good, but then I had this virus that attacked my heart and caused all the ensuing problems that I had.

I was lucky to survive. There's what's called an ejection fraction in your heart which is the amount of blood that comes into your heart and the amount of blood that flows out of your heart. I don't want to get too technical but my ejection fraction between blood coming in and blood coming out at that moment I had my stroke and heart failure was 15 per cent. A healthy person would be about 50 per cent. When I got the heart transplant in 2022, my ejection fraction was down to about 8 to 9 per cent, meaning you literally can't even get out of bed.

I had to get what's called a defibrillator. A defibrillator is like everyone remembers from going to school, or going to the airport, or going to a game. They have these paddles that they put on your chest, and they always say, 'Stand back.' It gives an electrical shock to get the rhythm of your heart back. So, imagine that inside my chest. Clearly, it's much smaller, but it's the same principle. There's a wire underneath my collarbone, and there's an electrical pulse that goes directly to my heart, and that shocks my heart back to normal.

So, I came out of the hospital with a defibrillator thinking that, when I got back to speaking, everything would be back to normal, but it was an ordeal to get back to normal.

I was so depressed, but at the same time I have a wife, two kids, and a business. I had multiple people working for me to produce movies, so it was like a little mini studio making one or two movies a year. When I lost that business, I was going through speech therapy, and I remember it was like I could hear people talking to me, but I couldn't communicate what I wanted to say. It was almost like being trapped inside your body with the inability to speak.

I remember going to speech therapy and the therapist was telling my wife (I couldn't even say my wife's name after months), 'I think that's the best it's going to get,' and my wife was totally heartbroken.

And I was thinking: who are you, who's this woman telling me what I can do and what I can't do? I wanted to rise above because I'm obstinate, and I didn't want to accept the reality that I'm not going to speak again. I wanted to prove her wrong.

At that time, it was so depressing, but you have to move on, there were too many people that were depending on me, and also I was a young man; I mean, relatively speaking, having this happen when you're 45 years old – well, it's the prime of your life. That's when you start making money from the fruits of your labour and I got struck down at that point in my life.

So, things progressed from there with tenacity, determination, and commitment. I wanted to figure out a way because everyone worries about money – and it's usually the lack of money – and money was running out. So, I had to kind of figure out a way to reinvent myself, even though I really was not speaking at that time.

There were the darker days and there were many where you just go into your mind and there's that voice that says, 'Am I going to make it?' You have all these doubts. And having the defib – I would say, even though I had a high stress tolerance to stress, it was the most stressful point of my life.

So, you're totally stressed out, you have to make money, you have to succeed, but at the same time you have these tremendous doubts. Can I do it? Can I put my head down and achieve it?

There were moments of thoughts about suicide. There were moments I was suffering from PTSD, you know, and that comes from when I first got sick, and from having the defib. One time I got shocked multiple times. The defib didn't work, so it shocked me again. Back-to-back. And then I was talking to my cardiologist, and I said: 'I'm fearful of going to bed at night.' I mean, I was tired, and I was thinking I'm gonna get shocked again and with all the drugs, the meds that they're putting me on, the cocktail of meds – you want to go to sleep. And it's not a good sleep. You wake up periodically and you worry, and you're stressed out. Am I gonna get shocked again? So, he gave me another drug to relax me.

* * *

So, yeah, it's been very stressful and with moments of suicidal thoughts and moments of depression. But a deep, deep, dark depression, with no ability to really explain it to your wife, your significant other, the person that is closest to you that you go to bed with at night and they're part of your team and they're your caregiver. You go into this world alone and you can't really explain how you're feeling because she wants you to say it's going to be okay. And you're thinking it's not going to be okay. And if you say it's not going to be okay, she panics and then the household panics and then you're trying to be the man of the house and not admit your own feelings. It was a very difficult period of my life.

I have developed my own philosophy about how to recover from the trauma in my life, and just to recap: I had a virus that attacked my heart. I had heart failure. I had two strokes. I got a defibrillator. I was suffering from PTSD. When I got the heart transplant, I had pulmonary oedema. I had aphasia – can't really speak. My ejection fraction was 9 per cent. It was just overwhelming.

I don't want to preach; I just want to tell you that what has worked for me is talking. There are voices inside your head. I don't care who you are. There is the yin and yang. There's like, 'You can do it. You can't do it.' And you have to compromise with those voices inside your head and hopefully work it out.

My philosophy I practise every day. It's not like I do it once a week or every other day. Every day. And it sounds horrible but *meditate*. You know, it sounds hokey, but it's just relaxing. It's just deep breathing. So, I do that for two minutes in the morning, and eight minutes at night. I like to get up, two minutes in the morning, before my shower. Just focus. What do I want to do? And then I exercise. I walk. I believe in having a purpose. Do you have any chores? Because you can't just wake up and have no purpose in your life. So, I've got chores. I have to walk my dog. I have to do certain things. So, I walk. And I walk a lot. I walk about 10,000 to 15,000 steps a day. Then I work out at night. I work out for about an hour, you know – mind, body, and spirit. I've heard this for my entire life, but finally it's sinking in.

So, I walk. I work out every day. I control my anxiety because anxiousness causes stress and stress invades your body. Stress causes high blood pressure, and the high blood pressure has consequences for your heart. It's the same thing.

Whether you have a gambling addiction, sex addiction, shopping addiction, whatever your addictions are, you have to control them. Listen to your body. Forget your doctors. Forget everyone that is around you. You know your body better than anyone else. Because your body is sending you signals like 'I can't feel my foot' and I make a note. Whether it's in your calendar or your smartphone, make a note: 'Okay, right now, I've got floaters in my eye. This is new. This is new because of the drugs I'm on. I've got three immunosuppressant drugs I'm on. One of the side effects of this drug affects my retina. And the retina, I don't know for sure, causes floaters in your eye. Never had that before, but I know there's a root cause.' So, listen to your body.

And don't abuse your body. Some people need whatever drugs or narcotics, but just try to be smart. That's what I try to do.

But the simplest things are almost the most complicated because it's so simple you can ignore it. Don't ignore it. Don't ignore your body. Don't ignore exercise. Don't also ignore the food that you put into your body. They all help you survive.

When you're younger, is it fair to say that you don't really think about this? You don't think about what you're putting into your body. You don't think about what you eat and how much you might drink, alcohol or drugs. A lot of things that we do to our body and our mind when you're inexperienced, you don't know what the effects are. However, the beauty of life is that when you fight those compulsions and feelings, when you fight that depression, when you fight those suicidal thoughts, you can get back to normal or relatively normal.

The thoughts go through your mind, but then you have a chance to make over. Every day is a chance to make it up. Everyone, when you fight with your friends, your siblings, your spouse, or your kids – you're mad at that moment. The next day, the sky is still there. You know, you have a chance to do it over again.

* * *

In 2021, my defibrillator shocked me twice again. I was rushed to hospital, and I was given a new heart in 2022. First of all, clearly, it's a used heart. Everyone says it's a new heart. It's not new; it's a used heart. And used hearts have problems themselves.

It's almost like an out-of-body experience. You're in the hospital waiting for them to call. Someone's going to tell you – you get a new heart. You're just anxious to get that new heart. And then the call comes in. You're getting a heart today, not getting a heart next week, because next week – we don't know what's happening next week. All we know is you're getting a heart today and it's surreal.

And then it's really real. Today, they're going to cut open your chest. For me, it was a nine-hour surgery, and I got a new heart. It was a female; it was a woman's heart. So, interestingly, because I'm not a big guy – I don't weigh a lot: just to put it in perspective, I'm 5'7" and I was 120 pounds – so that size could work for a man or a woman. So, they gave me a woman's heart. I thought the hard part was getting the heart and then they adjust your meds. But the hard part for me was the after-effects of getting the heart. The woman that I got the heart from had dormant problems in her heart that I now had. She's the donor. I got her heart and whatever's wrong with her heart, I inherited.

She had what are called spasms. It's usually for a second or two seconds or three seconds. So that means, first of all, I was in the hospital two weeks, and they didn't know what was going on. And the heart spasms were really active. The cardiologist looked at my chest because he thinks it's made up, because it doesn't show up because it's so instantaneous and it doesn't show up if someone is not watching the monitor. So, he puts his hand on my chest, and he said: 'Oh, I get it. Your heart is spasming and it presents like you're having a heart attack.'

Having said all of this, I'm just thankful I have a replacement heart, so I don't really care that much that it is a donor heart. Before getting the heart, I just thought I was doomed. Literally my heart was not pumping, I had fluid on my lungs, so I was going to die. All my cardiologists – and my surgeon – said: 'You're at death's door.'

So, I recognised that. And then I got the heart in August 2022. There's a moment of joy and then the reality is that you get all these problems with the donor's heart and that is now a part of me, so I got so depressed. I mean, why me? I mean, I've had all these problems. I thought I was a healthy person. I got strokes, heart failure, couldn't speak, then I got a new heart. And then, you're so upset that you're the only person in the world that is having all these problems, so you have to kind of get out of your own mind. My sense of humour was almost like gallows humour, you know – it could be worse. I don't know how much worse, but it could be worse.

* * *

They offer you an opportunity to write a letter to the family of the donor heart, and originally my letter was: 'Oh my God, I got a heart. Thank you so much.' It was like the ether in the air, the drugs in the air, because I got the new heart in that first month. However, I waited a year just to see and my view changed. So, in the end, I thanked the family for the heart, but I was not overly enthusiastic. I was a little more couched in the way I expressed myself. But it's you – this is happening to you; your depression is happening to you; your moments of like, 'I'm going to commit suicide' are happening to you. No one else. But you have to pause and then take a deep breath and then, you know, tomorrow will be better. You have to have some optimism, because it's so dire. But at the same time, will the sun come out tomorrow? Would the sky be there tomorrow? These are such basic, stupid things, but you go through these emotions and then you conclude, yeah, it's better in a couple of weeks, but at that moment, it's so oppressive – but you have to get through it.

I feel gratitude for lots of things in my life, which I never thought I would. I was a taker, you know – whatever I can take, I'm going to take. I didn't really have a lot of gratitude, but today I think about how grateful I am for certain things, how grateful I am to have a family, my wife, how grateful I've gotten friends that can keep me grounded; you have to make sure of your support system.

How am I doing today? There have been lots of problems with this heart, but right now I'm so happy to be alive. I feel I'm doing great. If you look from the outside, I'm looking great. I'm feeling good, although from the inside it can sometimes be a different story.

But you know, I've always beaten the odds. I have to be more optimistic and what will be will be. I mean, I don't know what the future will be. You just have to deal with it day by day and find optimism in your life that you're grateful for. And I'm grateful that I'm telling my story and feeling good.

I don't want to be a victim of circumstances. Like, you know, people pour these things onto you: 'Poor me, poor me.' And you're a victim of circumstances. All these things, extraneous things, are happening to you. I want to be more proactive but also patient – and literally I have been a patient. But you also have to have patience that things will get better – and, you know, sometimes they get worse before they get better; there's an ebb and flow to life. There's an ebb and flow to your health. There's an ebb and flow to your relationships, so I feel that, being a patient of circumstances, I have taken back control of my life – not being a victim. Be patient and things will get better in the future – that's what I feel.

Life is a tragicomedy, so you have to look at your life when you're in the thick of it, step back and say, you know what, there is some humour in what's going on for me – there has to be some sense of humour, and there's irony in life and you have to mix that with optimism.

I've been at the lowest point of my life, depressed; and still, I go in and out of depression, but I'm not chronically depressed. I'm not getting suicidal thoughts any more; I moved on, but I'm still anxious. That's not going to change. But you do need to jump in the deep end, because the cold water will shock you. But at the same time, you're swimming – and you get warm. Every day you have a chance to do it again.

Sometimes, life can change in an instant. My life changed in an instant. It wasn't planned, but what you do next will define you. Not what you've done in the past, but what you're doing next.

Hopefully, some good will come out of my story and you'll say: 'My God, I'm glad I'm not him!'

OCTAVIAN
DIAGNOSED WITH ADHD AS AN ADULT

'I've been called lazy. I've been called unmotivated. I've been called superficial. Internally, I just didn't feel that way. I've wanted to be successful, to finish what I had to do and to show people that I'm worth it. I'm worth something. But I could just never finish anything or do the things that lead to success, unfortunately. For most of my life, I didn't know what was wrong.'

My name is Octavian Constantinescu – it is a long name – and I'm a business consultant from Ontario, Canada. I've lived here for about 26 years, but I was born in Romania, and I lived there for close to 14 years, which means that this year I'm turning 40, and that is the age for mid-life.

It's one of those things when you say ADHD – normally what people think about is what children struggle with early on in their lives or maybe as they're approaching adolescence. We don't necessarily really think about adults with ADHD, mainly because it goes undiagnosed in childhood and it doesn't go away when you're an adult.

I was recently diagnosed with ADHD at the age of 39. This happened after living pretty much over half of my life not knowing what was wrong with me.

When I was in school, grade school, high school, I could never really focus on studying. I would sit and read for 20, 30 minutes, and then I started just spacing out or tuning out or starting to play computer games. The things that I was studying were just boring to me and I didn't have any sort of interest in them, no matter what I tried.

My parents sent me to tutors. I had tutors in elementary school. I had tutors in high school, and that helped because the other person, the third party, is helping you to focus your energy and mental capacity on what you're studying. However, when I went to university, the tutors just kind of went away.

I could never find the motivation to go to class, so I flunked out. Then, eventually, after getting married, I had almost another tutor in my life. I was able to finish a four-year degree. My wife helped me to stay focused on the task at hand. Even if I was bored, I had that additional motivation behind me to get the work done. And throughout this process, I never really understood what was happening.

I thought I was just lazy or unmotivated or procrastinating, because this also happened at work. As soon as I started work, I started to find it difficult to finish my tasks, whether it was finishing them correctly, to a high quality, or in a timely manner. And that issue went on for years and years and years.

I've been called lazy. I've been called unmotivated. I've been called superficial. Internally, I just didn't feel that way. I've wanted to be successful, to finish what I had to do and to show people that I'm worth it. I'm worth something. But I could just never finish anything or do the things that lead to success, unfortunately. For most of my life, I didn't know what was wrong.

It doesn't make you feel great, because you don't want to do those things on purpose. From the outside looking in, other people would just think that I'm doing it on purpose; but from the inside looking out, thinking about my own experience, it wasn't something that I wanted.

It almost felt like I was in a prison or being forced to do something that I didn't want to do and that just didn't feel good to me, because I have a pretty high image of myself. I always felt like I was meant to be successful, or I was a mover or a shaker, or both.

The reality was that I was only skating by, whether it was at school, whether it was at work. So those two realities just never really coalesced. There is a lot of cognitive dissonance happening in my brain because of that.

It led to many bouts of depression and, of course, the anxiety that goes with this sort of situation when you're not delivering results that are expected is going to be through the roof. When you're not living or acting in accordance with your values because of your decisions – and one of my values is to provide quality results – that leads to the depression side of things. But at the same time, I also felt like success was almost owed to me without doing the things that lead to success and that I was meant for greater things.

Because I wasn't getting what I thought I was owed, maybe in terms of promotion or more money or these things in your career that everyone is searching for, I started to get bitter. Then I started to put a lot of my energy into chasing these results, these things that I thought that I was owed, because I thought that my happiness was tied to getting those things, to getting what I felt I was owed. I thought that I'd be so happy once I got what I wanted, so I linked my happiness, my joy, to the outcomes in my career. But it was like running on a treadmill.

Once you put all your energy into a particular outcome or a particular goal, or a particular area of your life, other areas of your life will tend to suffer because you're not putting in the energy in those areas.

So, the problem was that I started to ignore the people around me who I now realise were actually the key components of my happiness, not my career and the outcomes of my career, but the people around me, and I just ignored them for years. I ignored my kids, I ignored my wife, I ignored my parents, and my friends, and I put 99 per cent of my energy into being successful in my career with very poor results in that area. And then of course, very poor results in the personal side of things because I didn't dedicate any time or energy to it.

* * *

Thankfully, there was a turning point which came in August 2022. I had a mental breakthrough that actually followed a mental breakdown. That's the thing about these things; sometimes good things come out of bad things. So, I had a mental breakthrough that I'd never had before. And I realised that my family and my friends are the only contributors to my happiness, to my joy, to my fulfilment as a person, and as an individual.

And I understood that life is about the relationships that we have with other people. Good relationships have been researched and linked to things like longevity, happiness, and even career success, which was a finding from the Grant Study out of Harvard Medical School.

For those people who are not familiar with this study, and even the people who are, it is always good to go back and read the outcomes. It was a very comprehensive study and it's still actually going on after over 80 years, following the same people, throughout their lives, and figuring out what has led to their success and what has led to their failures.

What that study found is that good relationships are the top factor when it comes to longevity, happiness, joy, and success. Now when I realised that relationships are the key to happiness, to success, to joy, I actually started putting in my energy and started working on repairing the breaks that I had created in my relationships with the folks around me like my wife, my kids, my parents, and my friends of course. So that was the breakthrough, and it has been an upward trajectory since then. Of course, there are dips and things that happen here and there, but I'm in a much better place today than I was before August 2022.

The funny thing is that I didn't recognise that I needed therapy at the time because I'm the kind of person who thinks that I can always help myself. I have that sense of independence ingrained in me. It's unfortunate because we really need to use all resources that are available to us, the people that are available to us, for support, encouragement, and as an addition to our lives – because we can't do everything by ourselves; it's just not possible.

But then looking at the future, my wife suggested that I go to therapy. I agreed with her eventually, but not at first. When she said that I need to go to therapy, I replied to her along the lines of: 'Why do I need to go to therapy when I have you?' Because, in my mind, I thought therapy was just talking to somebody, getting out what's on your mind and then being free of it. That is not what therapy is about.

The other thing she said that was key to my decision to go to therapy was that, besides the fact that she's not a licensed therapist – she's a nurse, but she's not a therapist – she is way too close to me to give good advice. And of course, there's also the issue of burdening her with my issues when she's got her own.

This completely changed my mind. I realised that I was counting on putting my greatest burdens on her when she didn't deserve that. She has enough burdens of her own, whether it's work, whether it's the kids, or her own family. She doesn't need my burdens as well.

So, at that point, I turned to something that throughout my life I considered as a last resort, but it actually changed my life forever. And that thing is therapy.

* * *

So, at this point, I hadn't been diagnosed with ADHD. The road to the ADHD diagnosis actually began when my daughter was diagnosed with ADHD. My daughter's doctor sent us a questionnaire and I filled it out for her because at the time she was nine years old. I answered the questions based on what I observed my daughter doing and feeling and saying – based on what she was telling me.

As I went through that questionnaire, I realised that my own personal answers to those questions were very similar to what I was observing in my daughter and what she was saying, and that started the gears going in my mind.

When I started therapy, I was talking to my therapist about these answers to the ADHD questionnaire, and I asked her for advice about the best way to either get treatment or to find out coping strategies. She agreed at that point that my symptoms were pointing towards ADHD and first she recommended a book that was very helpful in just understanding ADHD. That book is called *ADHD 2.0*, by Edward M. Hallowell and John J. Ratey, and it's excellent in explaining what ADHD is at a much deeper level than I can explain, and it's also great for providing coping strategies for people who have ADHD and adding those coping strategies to their arsenal in addition to medication.

The key thing to understand about ADHD is that the disorder itself is not a behavioural disorder. It's not a mental illness. It's not a learning disability. It's not something that you can develop. There are ADHD-like symptoms that people can develop depending on how they behave and what they do, and this is linked to our high-speed society, having a phone in your hand all the time, never being bored, and things like that. So, there are behaviours that mimic ADHD but ultimately it is not behavioural; it's a developmental impairment of the brain's self-management system.

It's genetic, so if somebody in your family has it, it's very possible that you also have it. People with true ADHD have at least one defective gene that makes it difficult for neurons to respond to dopamine, which is the neurotransmitter in the brain that is involved with feelings of pleasure as well as the regulation of attention. So, when we feel intense joy, that's our brain reacting to dopamine. And when we're able to focus our attention on a task and complete it successfully, again, that's the result of dopamine's action in the brain. So, if you have ADHD, the brain is not able to respond as it should to dopamine.

If you are wondering whether you might be affected by ADHD, and perhaps you're showing symptoms of the disorder, there are adult self-assessment tools available. For example, there's the Canadian ADHD Resource Alliance website [https://www.caddra.ca].

* * *

So, after getting the diagnosis I started medication and, honestly, it's just like night and day. Whereas before, maybe I could focus my attention for about 30 minutes on a task, now I can go for up to six hours a day. I can stay focused on work tasks. I can complete them in a timely manner and to a good quality. And it's something that I just never experienced before in my life.

The thing about work is that you could be doing your best. You could be doing all your work assignments on time. You could have the highest quality in your work as possible, but at the end of the day you don't actually control your career trajectory. You can get fired even if you are the best employee at a company. But what was happening before is that I wasn't creating good work. It wasn't timely, it wasn't of good quality, but I expected the outcomes that sometimes result from doing those things properly, like getting a promotion or getting more money, and so on and so forth. And because I wasn't getting those things that I thought that I was owed, I was dissatisfied and unhappy.

Now, because I am actually satisfied with the quality of my work – I'm completing my work on time and I'm giving it 100 per cent and creating something amazing – work for me is no longer a source of unhappiness. I just feel fulfilled, joyful and happy because I'm able to do what I'm meant to do, what I need to do, very well. I'm still a little bit stressed sometimes. Don't get me wrong. There are always going to be stressors in a work environment; that's normal. It's just that the part of me that was always searching for recognition or reward when I didn't deserve it, now that part of me realises that the only recognition that I need is in doing the thing properly, is in completing the work. So, the things I'm doing at work are no longer attacking my self-image, because when I wasn't doing things properly, that was an attack on my self-image. And of course, you feel like you're depressed because of that, and anxious because you're not completing things well. But now my self-image is no longer under attack, so I feel safe to perform at my very best or as close to my very best as I can get.

I can say with 100 per cent certainty that the two things that have been the key to where I am today are therapy on the one hand and then an ADHD diagnosis and medication on the other hand. Without those two things, I would still be in that state of unhappiness, of just always searching for recognition in my work, in my life, and ignoring the people around me, but in reality never getting that recognition and just having poor relationships around me because of it. So, I am 100 per cent convinced that this is why I'm seeing these positive results in my life.

The funny thing about how this all works is that now my career is about helping organisations to create psychological safety for their employees so that their employees can start performing at their very best or as close to it as possible, because the key thing here is psychological safety. When we as humans feel psychologically safe in an environment, we tend to perform at our very best.

The problem is, of course, that in most environments and most work environments, even school environments, psychological safety is missing from the employer side. So, I can go to as much therapy and take as much medication as I can, but if my employer isn't aiming to create psychological safety in the workplace, my results are still not going to be as great as they could be.

However, organisations are starting to take steps to create psychological safety, and I'm one of those people who help organisations do that now – it's funny that it all came full circle.

* * *

Invest in your mental health, which is the main advice that I want to give. You cannot affect your work environment. It's not in your control. You cannot affect the way that people see you or react to you. The only thing that you can affect is your own actions. Because that is fully within your control, invest in your mental health in some way. It's imperative.

Start with your own mental health. There are three more parts to this advice. If you're finding right now in this very moment that you are struggling with something that's always the same thing, over and over, take a really deep look at it and just answer this question truthfully: is this something a source of happiness for me or a source of unhappiness? It could be your career, it can be personal relationships, it can be anything in your life that is a recurring problem, and just ask yourself: is this giving me happiness or unhappiness?

Now you might be thinking, 'Well, it's a problem, it's an unhappiness,' but that's not really true. Because I thought that my family was part of the problem but truly, when I actually took a deep look at it, I realised that my family is actually part of the solution. It's a source of happiness for me.

The second part of the advice is that, if whatever it is that's bothering you is a source of unhappiness, think about it. Do you think it's because you are not very good at it? You know, like maybe not doing great work or maybe it's because it's a negative environment that you're in. Then there's a few branching decision trees. If it's because you're not very good at it, you can delve into why and how to solve that. If it's because it's a negative environment, you can delve into why and maybe remove yourself from it. But the conclusion here is that you have to analyse the situation. You have to put the time into this.

You have to put the time into your own mental health and dig deep. This isn't going to cost you anything but time at this point. You can also engage with a licensed therapist to guide you through it, because that is what they do. They guide you through it so that you can arrive at the right conclusions faster.

And then finally, the third part of this advice: if there's something that is always a recurring problem in your life, if that something turns out to be a source of happiness, if it turns out to be a source of satisfaction or joy – like family turned out to be in my case – then figure out a way to stop struggling with it. I just accepted it and started doing the right things.

The feeling of rest that you get from the end of this struggle is extremely refreshing and it gives you so much more energy, and you're able to actually think about investing in your mental health. And you're able to get out of that state of fear and anxiety and almost fight or flight, so that you can do the next right thing. Instead of making choices that come from fear, you make choices that come from joy.

The problem is that when you are in that state of mind, the things that are obvious aren't actually obvious at all, because you are in a kind of survival mode, but it's psychological survival. It mimics the same symptoms of physical survival, but it's actually psychological. So, when you're in that situation, you tend to make the wrong decisions. And one of the first things is to get out of the mentality of survival. To get out of that cycle of fight or flight, and to think rationally and create a plan to go forward. So that's what I want to encourage people to do. Yeah, this might sound really obvious that you have to invest in yourself and do the right things, but oftentimes it doesn't feel like it's obvious, and oftentimes it doesn't feel like it's achievable – but it's extremely achievable.

You can get started on that today by analysing the source of your unhappiness. What is that something that is always bothering you? Go from there: seeking therapy, working with those around you, using your systems of support. You do have to put in the work, 100 per cent. Nothing comes without work. I can guarantee that.

————————

To contact Octavian, visit his profile at
https://www.linkedin.com/in/octavian-c/
or email him at oconstan@gmail.com.

TOM
RESCUING YOURSELF FROM CHILDHOOD TRAUMA

'If you have painful, hard things that have happened to you in your past, it's very much like an open wound. It's a physical wound and until you begin to dress it, it leaks out in ways like your behaviour or your attitude.'

I was always a writer and that's what I did professionally. With some success and then other times not. I was a journalist and then I was a joke writer as well. So, I liked telling stories and that was kind of what I did and that's what interested me.

On my upbringing, just to give you the background of it, my dad was a very violent man. Violent towards my mum. I had triplet sisters, and he was also violent to them and he led a reign of terror really over the household. I think the consequence was, although it all happened when I was a kid, I didn't tell anyone, because I'd have been betraying my dad in some way.

I also felt a bit of shame and didn't talk about it. It was definitely something that the whole family kept secret and I kept that all locked away for 40 years. When I started to think back to it and started to confront some of those things from the past, writing about it seemed the most natural thing to do for me.

I also sort of remember thinking, 'Well, hang on. I'm always sitting here thinking of stories I could write. This actually seems to be the best story that I've got.' Because like anything in life, it's just real. And it's like – you can't make it up, because there are too many twists and turns and strange recurrent themes that showed me it was a story that, really, I had to write and that was the best way into it for me – and a way of dealing with some of those difficult things in the past and confronting them through writing.

I think that there were two triggers for writing the book. My dad died, and I had a very complicated relationship with him growing up. You know, as a kid you want to be with your dad when you're three or four years old. He was a charismatic, charming man. He could be a lot of fun. So, I really wanted that relationship. But he had this other, horrific side, and he was a monster, and I couldn't really understand that as a child.

So, I just sort of looked to try and maintain that relationship and I never really looked at it and I kept that relationship with my dad all the way into adulthood.

So, I suppose my dad dying was a kind of semi-trigger in a way, because I was able to look at that relationship a bit more objectively without having him around.

The other trigger was when I looked at my son one day when he was about four years old, and that's when I had my first memories and remembered growing up in this violent house. So, when I looked at my son, I kind of started to think: 'What if he had seen the things that I had seen? What if the things that happened to me had happened to him?' And I thought it would break him in many ways, and I wondered if, perhaps, the things that had happened to me had broken me in some way.

So, many days would be kind of peaceful. We'd watch a film together. My dad and I played a game of chess. Just sort of normal activities that a family might do, but then he would have a sort of switch that would turn, and you never quite knew what it would be. It could be totally insignificant to anyone else, and he would be just become a madman and he would hit, punch, and kick my mum.

I know that he raped her too. He would drag her by her hair down the street while the neighbours watched. The police were called lots of times, but he had a real control over my mum. We were in and out of refuges so sometimes we got away. However, he had a way of getting my mum back. Living like that, I mean, you're just on eggshells the whole time, so even when there's peace it's not really peace because you're thinking what's going to happen next. And it was totally and utterly devastating because of the kind of fury that my father had – I've never seen anything like it in my life to this day.

It was a bit like a war zone, really. Not with bombs but there's never a moment of 'Ah, this is fine; this is okay.' So, you take all that tension; that tension is always there.

* * *

It's hard to remember how you thought as a child, but I knew that other people didn't have to contend with that at home. I'm pretty sure that because I was aware of wanting to keep it a secret, and the embarrassment of having the police called, it was the last thing I wanted to tell people. If I had to write an essay about my weekend, I wasn't going to write about that.

Our neighbours were aware of it, and maybe they called the police sometimes, but they didn't really do anything. I just kind of thought that everyone seemed to stick their head in the sand about it, and because my mum put up with it – and it was very, very difficult for her – I guess I didn't really look at it that way as a kid. I just thought: 'This is my dad and I wish there was a way that I could stop him doing this, but this is life, and you have to get on with it.'

And when these moments happened, me as a seven- or eight-year-old, or whatever I was at the time, had to find the best way of managing it. So, I spent a lot of time trying to control him, calm him down, manage him, standing in the way of my parents, and that is a huge obligation on a small child and especially one to take on themselves.

But of course, I didn't realise that at the time. I don't think my mum was really aware of it, because for her she was just in survival mode. You're not thinking of escaping because you're thinking: 'How do I get through today? Keep alive.' I think that was what my mum thought. And for me, I had to try and protect my mum. I looked at myself as a sort of bodyguard, but I was useless at the job because I was so young. All that I could do was to try and do my best to manage my dad's moods and to try and be awake so that when these arguments would be at night, or the violence would be at night, I could have some sort of small control over it.

I just longed for those moments of tranquillity where there was no violence, there was no fighting, my dad was in a good mood. That's what I was looking for. And I guess there was hope there that maybe this will stop eventually, maybe it might be a week or two weeks without any incident, and you think, well, maybe it could go longer than that.

As a kid, I couldn't break it down. This was my life. This was the man we lived with. Let's try and survive it. And I think it didn't go beyond that and then I think I got trapped later in life in that thought process. I would see stories on the news about domestic violence and horrific things happening and think 'How terrible for them', without relating it to the fact that I had been there myself. I knew it had happened. If I talked to my mum about it, we would say, 'Wasn't that an awful time?

I'm so pleased we're out of it,' and our conversations wouldn't really go beyond that to the effects of it, what it actually meant.

So, I sort of got trapped in that thought process, and I couldn't break it until he died and that kind of broke something, and then having my son slowly allowed me to think, well, what does it do to a child? Because you don't know that you are any different from anyone else.

But I was a tense person, and I had a lot of nervous energy, and I was ready for the world to explode at any moment around me, any situation. And I had to be ready to fight. And that's how I lived my life in this tension that I lived with all the time.

* * *

I was also very keen to protect myself from anyone asking questions about my past, and I think I didn't really want people to know me properly because there was this darkness inside that I hadn't worked out myself.

So, then I put on an act. I think this is what loads of people do, and we might all do it to some extent, but I just became this person that would tell stories, who was good at parties. I wanted to be really charming, and smooth, and when I was out I was just performing, and I think that that was the consequence for me. And until I looked at it, I couldn't untangle, unwind any of that mess.

Trying to understand my dad, I knew that he came from a violent home himself. His dad was violent with his mum, so he learned his behaviour first-hand from first-hand experiences.

And I think from things that he said himself, I think his mum was particularly horrible to him with punishments, and I think he had a lot of anger about that. Hitting him with sticks or whatever, or kind of humiliation, really. I think he was made to wear some sort of potato sack or something, and I think he was just a very, very angry man and he was intent on taking it out on people. He was a very violent man. He had lots of fights growing up and I think he repeated the behaviour he witnessed first-hand growing up.

You only have to look at lockdown and all the calls to domestic abuse hotlines to realise it's still very much real now, just as it was 20 years ago or 50 years ago. I think it's always happened, and sadly always will, until these things are much more in the public consciousness and we can talk about them and call them out.

Back when he was growing up in the 1950s, I think there were a lot of traumatised people from the Second World War, who may well have used violence as a kind of outlet for some of that trauma.

I think there was an understanding that an Englishman's home was his castle so what happened in there was his business. There's a kind of sexist attitude to it. I doubt the police would've been particularly interested. I know that even in the 1980s, when the police came to our house, it was always viewed as a breach of the peace rather than an assault. And the police would usually just go away. They'd ask if everything was okay, and maybe they'd detect that there was some sort of tension in the air, but they'd just have a word with my dad and they'd consider it job done. The police didn't have the training to realise that maybe someone is not going to speak up in that type of situation. I think that things are getting slowly better as we kind of educate ourselves, but I think it's just a problem that persists and carries on through generations.

* * *

Since writing the book, people get in contact and want to tell me their own stories that are either similar or have echoes of my story. People write to me saying 'I experienced something similar' or 'I grew up like this'. Maybe it was worse, maybe it was a one-off incident, but it deeply affected them. Of the people that I know who have read the book, I would say almost half of them have had some experience of domestic violence. And that shook me.

It just shows me how widespread this thing is. I mean, it's incredible. Everyone's got some sort of difficulty from their past that kind of haunts them in some way. I never knew this before because I've never involved myself in big emotional conversations with people in that way, or I wouldn't really listen to it because I couldn't really handle other people's pain without being able to handle my own. And it's only now, when I've got a grip on my own difficulties from the past, that I've been able to understand other people.

If you have painful, hard things that have happened to you in your past, it's very much like an open wound. It's a physical wound and until you begin to dress it, it leaks out in ways like your behaviour or your attitude. That was certainly the case with me, and I see it now clearly in other people in a way that I couldn't before.

* * *

We're all products of our childhood, aren't we? And when you have a disturbing childhood it's impossible to untangle these things as you go along without assistance or without help. So, for me, writing the book, I was able to spend time in those painful places and write and think about not just, well, this happened and that happened, but what did that actually feel like? What did it mean? What were the consequences? All those questions were incredibly useful in untangling the pain of the past and what it all meant.

I would always be really careful about giving advice about what people should do about their own traumatic pasts, but I know that if you don't, if you sort of block it out, it remains a bleeding wound. I'm sure that the only way is to understand the things that have happened and slowly come to accept them, and to do that I think you have to think as deeply as you can about them in a hard way.

And it's always frightening because it hurts physically to think back. I couldn't think back to my childhood. There were some images of me sitting on the stairs as a seven-year-old kid listening to an argument. That's how I think of myself as a kid. My legs shaking, sort of out of control, and I couldn't think about that moment without wanting to cry. And it was just too difficult, hard, and painful. But when I was able to write about it, start to think what it meant, how I felt on those stairs, listening to an argument, what did I need as a kid? Should I have been there in the first place?

When writing I could answer those questions, even if they were not particularly pleasant answers. No, I shouldn't have been there. I was alone. Understanding that, facing that, realising that, and then just accepting it. And that's what I had to do with my dad, really. Accept the good – there *was* some good in him, like everyone – and accept the bad and that it happened. The bad stuff happened, and it was shit, and that's what it was. But looking at it and examining the past in that way, for me, bought peace because otherwise it was just some dark shadow.

* * *

I used to have this thought of someone, like a sort of proper dad, rescuing that seven-year-old boy, and I kind of realised that there was no proper dad that was going to come. That's the truth. And actually, I had to rescue myself because I had to go and sort it out, work out that pain, and then I felt like I did kind of connect with that little boy that was me.

I had an image in my head of me as a little boy sitting on the stairs getting picked up and rescued, and actually I was the rescuer. I don't know if that makes any sense, but I was the one holding that little boy. It makes me very emotional even now because it's sort of the single most impactful thing; you rescue yourself because you have to.

And I think I found a way of repairing myself through my son in some ways by being the dad that I didn't have. And I knew what he needed because it was what I hadn't had. And through that relationship with him – he's eight years old now –

I do feel I've been able to give him all the things that you want as a child. And that's been incredibly restorative to me. And it's been wonderful to be able to give that.

....

Tom is the author of *Don't Ask Me About My Dad: A Memoir of Love, Hate and Hope.*

PAUL B
WHEN WORK HURTS: COPING WITH WORK-RELATED DEPRESSION

'So, I got myself off to my doctor, still not accepting that I was impacted by depression. Not at all, because I'm a professional person. I've got this wonderful career behind me with all this stuff I've done. I have a reputation, I have a profile, I have a personality.'

The first thing I must say is I don't present myself as being an expert in the field of stress, anxiety, or depression. My aim is really to share some of my own personal experiences and observations.

I'm nearly 60 years old and I grew up in Brixton, London. If I could look back at the five-year-old me on the streets of Brixton, there is absolutely no way I would think my life would turn out the way it has.

I've had to deal with some challenges in life, personally and professionally, but I've been very fortunate to have a really good career. I've travelled the world, and I've worked with some amazing people and now I have my own management consultancy.

So, you know, from an external perspective, I would say I've been successful. However, I will also say that success is not an antidepressant. Being successful doesn't mean that you're immune from the challenges that affect you as an individual.

I was initially in the military and then, when I left and went into publishing, that afforded me the opportunity to do a lot of travelling. Then I had a young family, and I decided to have a career that was based more locally within the UK. And as I went along, I worked in different sectors including financial services that were so not compatible with my personality – too aggressive, too cold – so, professionally and personally, I couldn't relate to it.

I left that and went to work in the public sector in a government-type organisation. And I thought, yippee, here we go, I can now slow down, you know, public sector compared to the private sector, less pressure. It will be easier. I can turn up and do a nine-to-five. I was in for a terrible surprise.

I went from being in very much a directional type of organisation, where you had profit as the focal point of success, to being in very much a collaborative type of organisation where service design and delivery was the measure of success. And I got very much involved in what I still do now, which is change management and transformation.

I first started to really feel the impact of being in a place which wasn't supportive of you as an individual when we were working on a major transformation project. It was over a period of about three or four years, and we were transforming everything. We had a turnover of about £1.2 billion and there were huge austerity measures in place. We had to take £250 million out of the organisation, and the impact of that was basically changing the way people work. It was cutting a lot of jobs. It was introducing automation. It was reviewing processes. It was large-scale disruption. And when you start to be involved in that type of environment, initially it's mentally challenging, but it's not difficult. But as time went on, the stress of doing that work started to play itself out into something that had much more of an impact.

I first started to notice something change because I could pride myself on being phenomenally sharp in meetings, and I think that was partially due to being younger as well, but I could walk into a meeting – I didn't need to bring a notepad or pen or anything – and I could literally sit in a meeting for an hour with multiple people there, listen to the meeting, engage, walk out and, a day or two later, still tell you exactly what each individual said. I was able to take in lots of information and analyse it and manage it without actually even having to take notes – it's just the way I used to be.

I started to notice a change when, one day, I was in a meeting – and this is probably a good few years into doing this particular type of work – and I went in with a notepad and I sat in the meeting and I was furiously taking notes.

So, something had changed; gradually I'd gone from this person who didn't need to take notes to now taking notes. I wasn't consciously aware of it, but I was furiously taking notes. And when I came out of the meeting, I looked at my notepad and I had no clue about what had just happened in that meeting. I was trying to recall what my action points were, what other people had done, and I had no clue, and I thought to myself: 'Oh my days, there is something seriously wrong here. What is happening?' And that became the start of me becoming consciously aware something was happening with my ability to function wholly competently in a work environment.

When I look back, I realise that the way that we were all working was just unreasonable. We're talking at the height of it – I would go three days, possibly four days, working through the day, coming home, having a short break, and then working on some form of documentation, working through the night, grabbing a small amount of sleep, getting up, going back into work, doing the same thing again, coming home, short break, working through the night.

And this was a constant pattern. And it doesn't mean that there aren't times in different types of careers where the urgency and importance of what you're doing may demand pushing yourself to that level. However, it should not be a consistent thing. Absolutely no way. And in this particular organisation, it became the norm. It was phenomenally toxic. I was part of an internal consultancy team. There were about six of us there. In the four years, we had nine different heads leading the team and we're talking about a role that was significantly senior in the organisation. People came in with their enthusiasm, 'I know how to do this', and then they saw the toxicity of the organisation. I recall seeing directors shouting and swearing at people publicly in the office. That type of behaviour should never be allowed.

A lot of the work I was doing was around technical transformation, so bringing in technology to transform how we deliver work. I would put business cases together, then develop programmes and project plans on how we're going to do it. We're talking multi-million-pound type of activities, and we're also talking about taking out a third of the employees that we had. There were about 9,000 employees, and when we finished the whole programme we were down to about 6,000. So, you're talking about taking a third of a workforce out, so there were big, impactful decisions that you didn't take lightly and that had to be really considered. If I was making a projection or implementing something that was going to remove somebody's job, I made every effort to make sure the decision was the best for the organisation and the person.

I'd produce very detailed technical documents, and they would be 50, 100, 200 pages long depending on what it was. You've got your summary document there, and the director will look at it, look at all the pages, and say: 'Can you get that onto two slides, please?' And you'd look at them and think, you know, even if you just read the summary and take the direction of the summary and not even go through the full document, you're about to make a decision that's going to cost your organisation a huge amount of money and change the lives of a huge amount of your staff. And you want it on two slides. That type of behaviour and that type of apathy among those leaders and the opinion makers created a very, very incompetent environment.

I recall that, once I became unwell, I was very much aware and sensitive to picking it up in others. And as much as we're talking about stress, anxiety, and depression, and it's seen as a negative, it's also a positive because it's almost like I've got an anti-depression radar. I can pick it up in others. I would ask the question 'How are you?' And they'd say 'I'm fine.' And I'd say 'No, how are you really?' And I'd pause and they'd look at me and they would know I've noticed them and their face will go very still. And then you see the change in their body. You know, generally, people start to curl up, their face will start to drop, and you could see the stress and depression. I can't believe some of the people who I thought were like really hard, stony-faced, and they were bursting into tears – and I'm talking about men here as well as women.

***

After I first noticed that my ability to function was impaired, there were other symptoms too. My sleep was terrible. I started to become less social. I'm a very sociable person and I just didn't have the energy to really go out and hang out with friends and do the things that I normally enjoyed. I think I probably at some point in time became quite short-tempered, you know; after a while it's just like you want everything to be done quickly. I'm quite a passive person, although I'm described as quite an alpha character, but I'm a very gentle person. I don't know how that works out, but my temperament became very impatient, and I found that I was constantly reactive, not just professionally, but it started to impact personally as well.

So, my enjoyment of life reduced. I didn't want to engage socially. Physically and mentally, I started to really, really feel it, until at some point I thought: 'Right, okay, let me reach out for help.'

The worst point for me was that I was absolutely exhausted. Out of the team of six of us – there was one lady and five guys – all of the men ended up being very seriously ill. One person – and I can't say it's due to the work, but I think it was a big factor – had a heart attack and died. Another one ended up with some thyroid or glandular-type issue. Quite serious. Another one's hair was falling out. And we were all healthy, fit people when we started, but we all developed different ailments.

Another factor is that I think sometimes we don't realise how much we define ourselves by our work. We may define ourselves in our relationships as being a husband, a father, a brother, a son, or whatever. But if those things aren't working very well – and for me, at that time, I was single, and those things weren't working well for me – work then became the defining factor for how I validated my self-worth. So, for me, if that suddenly stopped working, then how do I start to validate who I am?

And I remember going to the HR director and I said to her: 'Look, I don't know if you realise, but the team is struggling. We're under so much pressure.' And she said to me: 'Yes, the exec board has noticed and we're going to bring some help in.' And to repeat, being successful is not an antidepressant and it can mask the fact that you're putting yourself under a huge amount of pressure. I took some time off and I went to bed, and I didn't get out of bed for maybe two or three days, and I thought: 'What the heck is going on here?'

I think there's a point with depression where you are no longer in control and your body will say to you: 'Enough is enough; we're not doing this.' So, I got myself off to my doctor, still not accepting that I was impacted by depression. Not at all, because I'm a professional person. I've got this wonderful career behind me with all this stuff I've done. I have a reputation, I have a profile, I have a personality.

So, I went to see my GP, and I sat in front of him. He knew me very well and I said: 'Look, I'm really tired. I just think I've overworked a little bit, and could you just sign me off for maybe a week so I can get some extra rest?' And he looked at me and he said: 'You're not tired. I know you; you're depressed.' And I looked at him in horror and it was like a band-aid had been ripped off or it was like I was sat there naked and exposed. I remember stammering, trying to cover up my vulnerabilities: 'No, no, I'm not depressed, I'm just tired. We've got these projects and I'm working really hard', and I did everything I could to try and cover up what the doctor clearly saw. And he said: 'No, you're definitely depressed. You've been working like this for such a long time, and it is way too much and your body's telling you: time to stop. You need to be off for a minimum of three months.' I said: 'No, I can't do this. It's not possible.'

In my head, my doctor then became the person who's

coming to assassinate my career. It's like his words were a gun he's holding to my head, and he's now about to destroy my career. How can he say I'm depressed and give me that label? And three months? Are you crazy? What are people going to say? Anyway, we ended the conversation, and I said: 'Look, I just need a sick note for a couple of weeks and just say it was down to undue stress.' He wrote out the sick note and gave it to me and I left and went and sat in my car feeling really tired. I looked down at what he had written – I'm feeling quite teary right now thinking about this – and he had written *'suffering with depression, should not come back to work for 12 weeks.'*

I sat in that car, and I cried. There was a massive mixture of emotions. It's now out there, because I knew I couldn't go back to work in the state I was in, but I had to give somebody the sick note to tell them why I was off, and it actually spelled out what it was: *depression*. So, I thought that was the end of my career. The end of my life as I know it and I'll never be the same again. I'm useless. I don't know how long I sat in that car, but I can assure you – it was a long time. I couldn't drive. I just sat there and eventually drove home and I went to my bed, and I didn't get out my bed again probably for a week or so.

* * *

Having good people around you is really important. It's really, really important. I told two of my closest friends and they were very supportive, but it came to the point where I had to tell work. And I remember making the call to my manager. It was a manager who, at that time, must have been the fifth person into the role, and it's laughable now because that should have been an indicator to the organisation that what they were asking this team to do was too much. And I said to him, 'I've been signed off with, uh, um, uh,' and eventually I said 'depression' and he said to me, 'Okay, you need to look after yourself,' or words to that effect, the type of managerial talk you would expect from a manager who's just been told by the employee that reports into him that he's been signed off for depression. It was no surprise to him, no doubt because he could see what was happening to the team.

I think one of the things I learned is that when you are in it, you don't see what other people see. We leak a lot as people when we're going through things and so I realised that other people probably noticed my performance had dropped well before I did.

This manager said to me: 'Would you like me to put you in touch with somebody who has gone through what you're going through now?' And I just said: 'Yes, please.' That's all I could think of saying. And then that ended that call and at the point the phone went down, I just thought my life is over now and my professional career is done. Dead. This is what you get for trying too hard.

I was still in phenomenal denial. Although I had told my manager, the act of then sending in the sickness certificate probably took about another six weeks. I remember it took me ages because it was another confirmation that you are broken.

* * *

I remember one time I was out playing football – it was cold, it was winter – and I decided that I didn't need to warm up. So, I just got out there, kind of jogged for about 30 seconds, and then started to play football. And then I did a turn. And in my head, I heard a really loud sort of bang. And then suddenly, about two or three seconds later, I felt this awful pain and I hit the ground. I had snapped my Achilles tendon – literally just snapped it.

So, I went straight to the hospital, and they sorted it out and repaired it. I then had to wear this massive oversized boot for about six months, maybe a bit longer because it took a while to heal.

And here's the difference. Wearing that boot and having snapped my Achilles tendon – both professionally and personally, I got so much sympathy. 'Poor you, you've snapped your foot.' I'd get on public transport and people would get up and give me a seat. People were really sympathetic. They were really understanding. I had snapped my Achilles. They could see it. They could relate to it. But it's strange because stress, anxiety, and depression are way more widely impactful in society than a snapped Achilles. Yet, we get very scared very quickly when we say we've broken or impaired our cognitive ability.

We've impaired our ability to interact. We've put our minds under so much stress that our minds have said 'Enough'. We need time to stop, to heal – a bit like the boot I had to put on – and to repair. And I think we're getting a lot better now, but I think we're still quite cautious about discussing mental health, especially as men; it's crazy that we have to be so cajoled to go and see a doctor when there are issues affecting us.

I'm hoping that my experience will encourage other men to just have a conversation, even if it's with one person. Go on, you know, your life will not be over.

I would say you can't really overcome mental health or mental well-being issues alone. I think it's incredibly difficult. You do need supportive friends. You may need professional help, so accept it. Accept that you're not going to do this on your own.

* * *

So, my manager put me in touch with a colleague, John. When my manager said to me, 'Oh, do you know that John suffers from depression?', I said, 'John who?' I mean, there was only one John in the office and when he told me his surname I thought: 'Nah, no chance.' John was one of the most talented technical programme and project management professionals in the team of people that we worked with. He was one of the individuals that I would look up to in terms of just how quick and able he was at dealing with issues, dealing with people, coming up with answers, coming up with solutions. How the hell can he be depressed? There's absolutely no way.

So, he put me in touch with John, who then gave me a call and he said: 'Really sorry that you're going through this. I'm here to see what I can do to help. And just to let you know, you're in great company.' And then he rolled off a list of people, current and historical people, who suffered from depression. And what he did was to normalise the fact that you're not that special. You're not the only one. This is quite normal, especially among high-performing individuals.

He sent me a book and it was almost like a kid's book, really simple language, and it just told the stories of all these famous people who had suffered and lived with depression. He shared his story, which was not dissimilar to mine, where he became depressed, but now he lives with it. He knows that he's susceptible to future depression, so whenever he feels that things are too stressful or too difficult, he pulls himself away a little bit and manages it. He has a little bit of downtime and then comes back. Now, I never knew this at all. And I'd worked with this guy for a good while. So, getting professional help or speaking to someone like John, or friends and family, having somebody to talk to and normalise things, really helps.

I had a friend; his name's Jason, but unfortunately he died a few years ago. I absolutely loved this guy to bits. Every day he sent me a text: 'Hi Paul, how you doing? Just to let you know that I'm here if you ever need to call me.' And it would go on for weeks. For a long time, I couldn't respond to him, yet every day this text would appear, and he would get no response. Eventually, when I was able to respond, I thanked him and told him how much I really appreciated his texts. It meant a lot to me because it was a few people like that – that just kept me aware. I sat down with him one day and when I told him that, for some time, I wasn't able to respond to him, he said: 'I know you couldn't, but I needed you to know I was there.'

Sometimes, for those of us who are supporting people who are going through issues, you don't get a response, but that doesn't mean what you're doing isn't impactful. Sometimes, it takes your experience, empathy, and understanding to help somebody else along their journey.

As a result of this experience, I've had so many family and friends who have come to me and said: 'Oh, by the way, I'm going through *x* or my sister or my brother's going through *x* – would you talk to them?' And I would go and talk to them. And then they found it easier to open up to me because I've suffered from depression, and I can tell them about my journey.

Now I try to engage in physical well-being. I try to engage in music and art. I try to engage in things that keep the 'Paul personal side' awake and alive and vibrant. It balances off any stress from work, so, you know, my life isn't validated by my work experience. My life is about who I am as a person, and work then supplements that.

I've learned to be more compassionate with myself, and kinder to myself, and I think that's one of the things which I would encourage for anybody who's going through stress, anxiety, or depression. Be nice to yourself. Engage in some positive self-care. Treat yourself like you would treat somebody else who needed help.

You know, we talk about resilience and being resilient in the workplace. Resilience is not about being at the peak of your output and maintaining it. Resilience is about knowing when to ebb and flow. When to pause and pull back a bit so you can then do work at that peak again.

* * *

I think the signs of depression can be gradual. There's definitely a before and an after and the classic ones have got to be changes in your sleep pattern, excessive fatigue, appetite changes like you lose interest in food and you're not eating, or you do the opposite – you start eating everything and anything. Also, things like difficulty concentrating and making decisions. If it's becoming increasingly harder for you to pinpoint and make a decision and stick by it, start questioning yourself. You don't have to become too analytical about it, but just reflect: 'Is the environment I'm in positive or negative? Have I been in it for a long time? How long is too long? Do I need to take a break?' If you're finding that your motivation is low and your energy is low; if you start to feel overwhelmed by tasks which previously were manageable; if your work performance starts to decline; if you find that you start drinking more and you start to isolate or pull away from your colleagues – they're all good indicators and I would say: don't ignore them. Don't ignore the red flags. Find somebody you can talk to and just get a sense check.

In essence, depression is prolonged stress or prolonged anxiety to the point that you can't bounce back. Remember, you're not alone. People around you will, at some point in their lives, go through some form of stress, anxiety, or depression. It is just part of who we are. So, don't be embarrassed about it. It's okay not to be okay.

SIMON & GARETH
HAVING A CHILD WITH SPECIAL NEEDS: TWO DADS SHARE THEIR STORIES

'I needed to spend time talking to my wife, outside of the practicalities of everyday decisions such as which anticonvulsant to give, what adaptations to make to the house, or where we are going to put the lift. All those conversations happened because they were necessary … Somehow, we needed to make a conscious and proactive decision to speak about other things. And I think that's true of all parents. All those clichés of date nights; there's a reason for them.'

GARETH: Simon and I used to work together a long time ago. I happened to be in the John Radcliffe Hospital in Oxford with [my son] William, and I was walking down one of the corridors and bumped into him.

SIMON: It was just one of those chance meetings where I thought, 'There's a friendly face. I recognise you.' And we stood in the corridor and had a good catch-up. But the immediate bond, and where we have common ground, is that we were both dads to children with special needs. In my case, my daughter Olivia had sadly passed away by that point, but I could see that Gareth was probably attending one of many outpatient appointments with his son that were very familiar to me in my journey.

GARETH: Anybody that has got or has dealt with a child of any age with a special need means you immediately join a sort of 'superhero club' where you take on a special set of skills. I've got the utmost admiration for anybody that I've met who has a responsibility for dealing with a child with any form of disability or special need. Having been there, done that, and got the T-shirt, it makes you realise what these people have to cope with above and beyond normal life.

SIMON: And I think you kind of morph into this strange situation where there's a lot of unsaid things that are just known. You spot things that you just would never have spotted before or known anything about when you're not operating within a special needs world.

My story began with my daughter Olivia, who was born back in the summer of 2012. My wife and I decided to start a family – I'd got a stepson, who was six or seven years old at the time – and we got married a few years before and decided to have a baby. Everything was going swimmingly well until the point of delivery, at which point it went pear-shaped and Olivia was starved of oxygen at birth and had a very difficult delivery. It's not the journey that you ever expect or anticipate from the glossy world of having a young family and bringing a beautiful baby back home.

So, from our point of view, it was a very much a dark time. We spent the first few weeks in the hospital with Olivia. After having had a very traumatic birth, she was rushed away from us into a neonatal intensive care unit and given an MRI scan within a few days to try and determine the effect of the oxygen starvation. We were sat down about seven days later and told the results of the MRI and that they'd found something they weren't expecting to find, that her brain had not been formed correctly during the pregnancy and that she would be severely disabled and life-limited and probably unlikely to reach her first birthday. That was quite shocking news for us to have to take in.

From that point forward, we were in uncharted waters and it was not what we were at all expecting. We had to adapt all aspects of our lives. We're pretty competent people but we felt we were sent home without any real support or direction other than just 'Go home and enjoy your daughter,' and to get on with it. When the first health visitor came into our home, she didn't have any knowledge that we'd had a difficult birth and was as shocked as we were at what had happened. Going through those first few months was hard, having to adapt to life around a baby that needed extra care with feeding and all sorts of aspects. Life was just not normal in any way, shape, or form. We both had taken time out from work and had been supported by our employers to just do what we needed to do really to steady the ship. But it wasn't until about 12 months later that we got some form of social care support or referral to any kind of service.

By this point, we had converted the front room into a bedroom so that one of us could stay up with her through the night to help with feeding. She was being fed through a nasogastric tube, she was having seizures, and so on. And it was then a journey of referrals through various specialist hospitals, trips down to Great Ormond Street in London, genetic testing, all sorts of stuff that was being investigated. We found out she was blind. She had difficulty swallowing. All sorts of things that just unfolded as this journey went along. It was a very stressful time, as you can imagine. I was trying to work remotely, but caring for a child that needed so much of my time and attention took its toll.

It culminated in me having a heart attack in November 2013, which was pretty much a low point for us. Me in hospital, my wife at home having to cope with everything. And it was at that point that we got a referral into what we now know was sort of continuing care, which was where we should have been referred much earlier, in my view. But it meant that, because we were having to cope with acute episodes of care, we had open access to the local hospital, which meant we had unplanned admissions where we'd be going in and trying to do everything we could just to keep the wheels turning.

My wife also suffered ill health. She suffered from epilepsy. She'd had a seizure earlier that year. She couldn't drive. It meant I was doing all the legwork in terms of getting to all these different hospital appointments and moving my sort of mobile hospital ward that Olivia became with us wherever we went, so it was tough.

I suppose it was probably then after another year of just sort of trundling along like that, starting to get a little bit of better support for her, then realising that she had made it past a year, and at this point she was nearly coming up for three, and wondering what life was going to look like.

We needed to adapt the house. It wasn't suitable for Olivia's needs, and we needed to make sure that we had an environment that could provide short, medium, and long-term care for her. We couldn't get her upstairs. She was too heavy to lift. We had no specialist equipment in the house, so we took on the challenge of adapting our house. We moved out into a rented property for six months while we gutted our property to build a bedroom, wet room, and utility room, putting in a hoist, putting in a rise-and-fall bath, making it a spacious area, levelling out what was previously steps and making it wheelchair-friendly, and so on.

We moved back into our house, and I think it was by this point we'd got a better care package now arranged through the social care programme that we were part of with the local authority. We were getting continuing care support, which meant that we could have overnight care. Carers would come in at ten, go at seven, five nights a week, which was brilliant because it meant we just got a basic night's sleep, and we didn't have to worry about Olivia with her different medications and all these kinds of things that we were going through. It was a heck of a journey.

Through various DNA testing, it turned out that Olivia had a genetic mutation. It was a never-recorded genetic mutation – never seen before, never seen since as far as I'm aware – so she was a unique little girl in that respect.

I suppose what amazed me was just how uncoordinated the whole journey was, with none of the services really talking to each other, and it kind of fell to us to keep tabs on what was happening and what was available to us from sourcing equipment, wheelchairs, vehicles, to specialist seating, you name it. We had to kind of pull the whole thing together ourselves.

You have to just acknowledge that life is going to be different for you and it changes all aspects of your life, quite honestly. My wife wasn't able to go back to work because she took on the role of full-time carer. I was very fortunate in that I worked for a large company that recognised the unique situation I was in and gave me the flexibility to work remotely. I know that's what we all do now, post-Covid, but then it was good of them to do that and to support me. I'd been an employee of the company for quite a number of years, so they recognised that, and it meant working odd hours to fill in what I could at whatever times.

But all aspects of our lives were put on hold, quite frankly, because everything was geared around the care and support that Olivia needed. In the 12 months preceding my heart attack, we were just battling on our own with no real care or support from anybody outside. I suppose it almost felt like we were seen to be coping, and there were problems in the way that the different agencies didn't connect and didn't refer us. Maybe people had visited us in the home and thought, 'Yeah, they're coping, they'll be okay,' because, you know, British stiff upper lip – we just got on with it. But in reality: sleepless nights, stress, anxiety, worry, uncertainty about the future, uncertainty about adapting the house. Are we going to move? Do we need a bungalow? What are we going to do? Everything was up for review and debate, and I think it just took its toll, quite frankly.

GARETH: There are so many parallels. My starting point was slightly different. The birth was horrific – and that's as a spectator; I wasn't actually involved in the physical trauma of it all – but it still was, and I think that is true for a lot of people.

After a couple of weeks in hospital, with treatment, William was discharged and came home. He struggled to feed from the outset, so we battled with feeding, which was the biggest issue really at that point because his brain wasn't well formed. There were a lot of things that in hindsight we just didn't recognise or didn't know.

At five months old, if you look back at pictures of William, he was so small, so thin. He was clearly malnourished, and he had 'failure to thrive', so was under a general paediatrician. Then he started having what are called infantile spasms, which are a form of seizure. They present in a certain way, and I could spot one a million miles off now, but they are very difficult to describe. We actually diagnosed them from watching a YouTube video and emailed the doctor, who agreed and told us we needed to come in and see neurology immediately.

We had all this stress building up from William not being able to feed or gain weight and having to weigh him constantly. There was a lot wrong with William and it was visible in hindsight, but at the time we were just fighting through it.

With the infantile spasms, you start getting into a treatment path in neurology. The diagnosis right from that point was really not very good and you start moving forward. At this point, William was still a baby, and the world's relatively well equipped for a baby. Then, as he started getting older, we were trying to consider ahead of time what he'd need in the future, but we didn't find out until later that there was only one other person that had the same genetic mutation that William had. So, we didn't know how the world was going to look for us.

We didn't know whether William was going to have a very short life or whether he would live a long life. We knew it wasn't going to be normal. With a lot of conditions that are more commonly understood, they follow a path, within reason, and you know what the future holds, but this simply wasn't the case with William and that was really hard to cope with.

Navigating the system is a full-time job, without any question, and there's an awful lot you don't know, but you don't know that you don't know. So, you form bonds and groups and have conversations with other parents living in this ecosystem. Your network is spawned out of all these interactions from hospital appointments, hospices, or school – and you learn from all of those people. But there isn't really ownership of you or your child from a health, social care, and education perspective. All of those are just disjointed and you have to own and navigate all of that – and you're not an expert in any of those things. So, it's really difficult.

I think, to cope with it all emotionally, I definitely threw myself into the practicalities of solving the problem that was immediately in front of me, and I think that was my coping mechanism. It's quite a functional coping mechanism. Then afterwards things catch up with me and I reflect on them, and I've learned better to cope with that. Stress no doubt has a huge impact on you and your relationship. My wife's hair started falling out, not quite a heart attack or seizures, but it took its toll. And that's in itself quite hard to recognise because all of your focus is on William, trying to work out what to do, how to do it, what to do best, and you neglect all else because of that. I think after a while, and William's now coming up to eight, you have to evolve that, and we've had more children, so you reflect on that and become better at it. But the problems are still there. It's still difficult to cope with and it's still difficult to understand your situation fully and how you need to manage it. But definitely, the practicalities are something you can own; you can take hold of them, and you can do something about them. But actually, as much as they're necessary, they're a very small part of the overall well-being of you and your family and the child that you're trying to care for.

SIMON: During our journey, I met other families through different services that we were linked to from different organisations, and for me personally I took it upon myself to introduce myself and go and talk to some of these other parents and just form friendship groups out of that.

I was quite lucky because locally, within a relatively small geographic area, there were three or four other families that were on a similar pathway to us. Some with slightly older children, some with slightly younger, but I wish I'd done that sooner in my journey. Probably, if we'd been referred to some of the services at an earlier age than 12 months, there would have been an opportunity to link up quicker and sooner to people.

It meant that we formed our own dads' social group, and we would meet up once every month or two for a catch-up. It was never more than a beer and a bite to eat, but it was good to meet like-minded people who were experiencing the same sort of challenges that I was as a dad and as a family. I just wish I'd met them a bit sooner. They were a great source of information, both in terms of the practical stuff which blokes are always pretty good at – you know, give me a problem and I'll fix it – but also in terms of how they were coping in their relationships with their respective wives and girlfriends and the impact it was having on their wider families. It's the old adage: you just need to get out there and talk to people. It just was an informal thing, and I used to thoroughly enjoy the interaction, and I got a lot from it.

GARETH: I think the world that you're trying to navigate needs to be better orchestrated by somebody in a professional sense. You end up having to be responsible, even for things that seem trivial to most people, like what equipment you need and all of those things. What ends up happening is you learn from other people within your own social group and then you take that to the professional, be it an occupational therapist or a physiotherapist, and say, 'What about this?' And then they typically go, 'Yeah, that makes sense.' But the onus is on you to do that. The only way you find that out is from other people. I think that the social group is really important from an emotional point of view and just an understanding point of view.

SIMON: From my point of view, I would strongly urge anyone in our situation to meet other parents and carers. Look around you and find families with children in a similar environment, and just build that informal network. That's where you get your best resource. That's where you'll find your most important allies who can share their experiences – good, bad, or indifferent – and learn from that. And don't be afraid to share your own journey. I was more than happy to open up from a practical point of view and share my journey with other chaps who were in this particular group. We hosted them on a building site, when we were in the middle of our building works, because some of them were about to commence on a similar journey and I thought, if I'd had the opportunity to do that myself, I would have really welcomed it.

GARETH: I think talking about your own experiences and your own story is a very important thing for the people you're talking to, but also for yourself, without any question. I think there's a degree of catharsis that comes with that process.

I would also say that, whether it's a therapy conversation or a non-therapy conversation, certainly for me it is important that you take time out, reflect, and spend time talking. I needed to spend time talking to my wife, outside of the practicalities of everyday decisions such as which anticonvulsant to give, what adaptations to make to the house, or where we are going to put the lift. All those conversations happened because they were necessary and it was only later on that we both recognised that I approach things very differently from how my wife does – not rightly or wrongly, just very differently. And so, somehow, we needed to make a conscious and proactive decision to speak about other things. And I think that's true of all parents. All those clichés of date nights; there's a reason for them. It's harder in my experience to do that when there are so many things that need to be done, that it can take away from the opportunity or at least the headspace to be able to actively have those kinds of conversations and work on yourselves and your relationship and everything else, outside of the battle that you're fighting day in, day out, just to get by.

* * *

GARETH: I definitely think there's a distinction between men and women and I don't know whether it's a reflection on me or whether it extends out further afield. I think that the network that Simon talks about happens more organically with mothers. Those bonds and that social network just happened a lot more easily for my wife. As a male, or maybe it is just me, I did deal with things differently and just threw myself into the adaptation of our home, which was an absolute minefield. It was such a big project for us. We've got an old house, and we had to build an extension so we could put in a lift and adapted bathrooms, put in a hoist, bought a wheelchair. There was so much going on I just jumped on it and really owned those things, because I could do the research and I could just get on with it.

We just kind of had this separation of duties and I didn't necessarily look out for the social side of things, or network in the same way, because I just threw myself into another aspect of it and we didn't join up necessarily in the middle as naturally as we needed to.

SIMON: Unless you're living our experience, we found that a lot of people didn't understand and thought Olivia would get better. Surely, they can fix whatever this is and surely there's a cure. The complexity of our particular case, and how the journey unfolded, meant that this was life-changing for us, and we had to adapt to it. Our social life changed for sure, but in a good way. It took us to a different set of people who could relate more to what we were going through, and we formed some good, strong relationships. So, you've just got to find your tribe.

* * *

SIMON: The decision to have more children was probably one of the most stressful things that we went through. The situation we found ourselves in with Olivia and being told that she was life-limited meant that, ultimately, we were not going to have the outcome we were expecting. So, we thought about this and decided that we wanted to try for another baby. We knew there was a risk because of the genetic malformation that Olivia had.

We had various tests and went for consultant-led care and were lucky enough to fall pregnant fairly quickly. It was very much a conscious decision that we wanted to go on and have another child.

We were fortunate enough that our daughter Jessica was born in the summer of 2015, so Olivia was still around. It was a successful natural birth and a completely different experience from the one that we'd had a couple of years earlier with Olivia. Jessica was 15 months old when Olivia sadly passed in October 2016, but she remembers her little sister. There are plenty of memories of her around the house, as you can well imagine, and all of those milestones and things that Olivia didn't reach we now live through Jessica, and she's absolutely delightful. So that was the best decision we ever made.

GARETH: With William, we did something very illogical. We were fortunate that we had some results from the 100,000 Genomes Project [which sequences genes and studies the role they play in health and disease], which was happening at the same time as we were thinking about having our second child. We were thinking about whether we could give William the care that he needed as well as care for another child and we went through complex scenarios trying to work it out. It ended up that with William there was a very rare mutation, and it was almost certainly not going to happen again, although there was no certainty. The risk of having an amniocentesis test was far higher than having a repeat of William's condition, which was almost impossible – or that was the understanding we had at the time and the way that was presented to us. However, despite knowing this, we still had the testing because the consequences of having two people like William would make it practically impossible for us to care for both effectively. And then our second child, Beatrice, was born.

We then didn't want Beatrice to only know life with William. We thought a neurotypical sibling would be good. So, we went through the whole thing again and we had the testing again with the risks associated with it, and everything was fine as you'd expect it to have been if you'd have followed the data. And then Charlie was born.

All's well because it ended well, but it was a very stressful and difficult decision to take for us both. And then now it's fabulous. The children are amazing. William has seizures every single day, sometimes hundreds in a day, but they just get on with it. They understand it really quickly. They are way smarter than we often give them credit for, and I think they bring a healthy dynamic to our family and all of our relationships. William, his parents, his siblings – all of us together are better off because we did make that decision. But it was a very, very difficult decision to take at the time.

I think, in general, kids are just great with kids with differences and disabilities. Parents will look strangely at William and not necessarily engage or ask, whereas a kid would come up to you and we'll be feeding William, putting food in his feeding tube, and ask, 'What's that?' And you go, 'Oh, it's a bit like a straw because he can't eat with his mouth,' and they'll just be like, fine, understand that, and move on, and adults just don't do that.

* * *

GARETH: One of the responsibilities I took on was feeding William, which was really not as straightforward as most people would think it is. William was given his first nasogastric tube when he was five months old, and at that point we were in a very dark place, moving from appointment to appointment, specialist to specialist – the list was endless.

We knew that we were not able to feed William orally, and we were given a load of formula feeds. Later he had a gastrostomy, which made it a little bit easier, which is a tube that goes straight into his stomach and a pump, and we were just told how to use all of this stuff and that's what William was going to eat for the rest of his life. And at the time it was just a fait accompli, you know, here we go. This is how you do it. This is what enteral nutrition looks like. And we went home and started that process and got used to it.

But William had all sorts of problems with gastrointestinal side effects; he had diarrhoea as well and was constipated on occasion. He had terrible reflux, which is just vomiting all the time. And that had consequences on his overall health and everything else – and this carried on for a while. We didn't go anywhere without a bucket because William would be vomiting into it. I remember that was a moment of realisation for me when I was taking delivery of boxes and boxes of this formula, and you look at the ingredient list and you wouldn't eat it. You just wouldn't go anywhere near it. If you're having it for every meal, every day for your whole life, it's got to have huge consequences. We're told how important a well-balanced diet is and lots of fruit and veg and all those things, which is without doubt true, but that just switches if you're requiring enteral nutrition. So, forget everything that we all understand to be a healthy diet and you're now having this ultra-processed formula and artificial nutrition for everything.

I just thought this doesn't make any sense at all, that there must be something else. I did some research, and I found out about this idea of a blended diet, which is where you take normal food, and you just blend it. It's as simple as that. Well, it's a bit more complicated than that, but the world had not really cottoned on to how much this group could benefit from real food, and people were just following this medical diet. So, we did a lot more research. We spoke to our dieticians, our speech and language therapist, and paediatricians, and they were relatively supportive, although not everyone.

Then we started William on a blended diet and almost overnight he improved his reflux. He found movement. Everything just got better. And he was just better. He looked better. He was healthier. His weight gain was better. But there's an awful lot of work that goes into doing a blended diet. You've got to get the viscosity right, you've got to calculate nutrition, you've got to make sure that you're feeding a healthy diet. Volume tolerance is also difficult if you've never eaten food, because you're not weaned like a baby.

The change in William was so dramatic that I became very evangelical about the benefits of it and was talking about it to anybody else who was in a similar situation to us. And I decided, because it's difficult and because there isn't enough in the way of resources to support people doing it, somebody needed to do something about it, and they weren't, and so I decided that we were going to do it.

I stood in the kitchen and had a conversation with my wife, just saying this is what I think we need to do about it, and clearly she had seen the benefits and everything that happened in William, just as I had. And it was one of those things where it got out of hand. We spent a lot of time and effort doing research, engaging professionals, building effectively a business, spending hundreds of thousands of pounds, and getting investors to help us and partners involved to enable us to bring out a product that was fit for purpose, and the resources and network behind it to provide information, and then tell people about it.

It was an awful lot of work, and it still is. But the feedback that we get is overwhelming. It's making the same difference to hundreds of people like us, and that number is growing all the time. And I think in hindsight sometimes people say, 'If you knew how difficult it would be, you'd never have started it.' That's definitely not the case for us. And we didn't know how difficult it was going to be. We didn't know how hard it was going to be and how time-consuming, but the benefits are overwhelming and we're helping so many people. It's something I'm incredibly proud of and it's named after William as well: Wilbo's Blends.

So now William sits and has a Christmas dinner with us. He eats with us all the time and sits at a table with his siblings. That's really important. He has a birthday cake that is blended up and he has it like anybody else would.

NICK
THE TRAUMA OF SUICIDE: THE PARENTS' PERSPECTIVE

(By his parents, Sue and Tim)

'So, I guess the moral of our story is that suicide can affect anyone. It doesn't have to be someone who's down on their luck. It can be someone who's at the pinnacle. It's just a mental health condition and, unfortunately, we lost our son.'

SUE: We're just a normal family. Tim and I met when we were younger, in our twenties, and after courting for a little while we got married, and on our first anniversary we discovered that we were going to be welcoming a baby, and Nick entered our life nine months later.

TIM: I graduated from the University of Illinois in January 1977, and Nick was born in February. And so, from there we moved back to Toledo, Ohio, which is where we're from. Nick, he was quite a guy. He had a spark; he was a spark plug. He attended grade school at Ladyfield, which was run by the sisters of Notre Dame, a Catholic school. There were a lot of highlights, but the biggest in our mind was when he played Scrooge, in his eighth-grade year. He practised the English dialect, and he was phenomenal – an amazing performance. He was a very good student and a very good athlete.

Nick then went to another Catholic school in Toledo called St Francis, where my other two sons later went – and it's also where I went. And I guess the highlight there was that he received the Oblate Award [the Oblates are a religious order with ordained Priests and they run the school] which is an award for basically the overall number-one student as far as academics, and he also won the athlete award. He was a great football player and a great wrestler. He really had the whole package.

SUE: I guess you would say he was an old soul because he spent a lot of time with people, and people came to him, and he shared himself with them. He was kind of for the downtrodden.

One of his very good friends was a young man who had some issues, who later passed away as well, and Nick was always there for him.

He did well in grade school. He did well in high school. He was a spitfire, I'll tell you that – he had a lot of energy. In fact, I can remember one time going to the doctor saying, 'I'm not sure if he's overactive,' and he said, 'Well, does he sleep? Does he take a nap? If so, he's just a normal boy.' He was our first child, so we were learning as we went along.

Then we had two more boys, so it was a very exciting and busy time. Lots of sporting events and all three of the boys were good students. That was our early life, I guess.

TIM: From there, Nick received a scholarship to John Carroll University in Cleveland, but he really wanted to go to Notre Dame in South Bend, Indiana. He got on the waiting list and, to be honest with you, he was somewhat devastated. He felt like he'd worked so hard and should have gotten accepted. He could have gotten in, in his second year, but by then it was like 'all or nothing' with him.

So, he goes to John Carroll – this is 1995 – and he's playing football, and he's doing real well, but he was saying he's homesick. Cleveland's only two hours away but in the summer of 1996, when he went back to start football, he came home and wrote us a letter to say he's dropping out. And we were like: 'Oh my God, what?! This all-American kid is dropping out.' So, we met with his football coach, and he said, 'You know, something's going on with Nick.' That was our first red flag.

* * *

TIM: So, after we got over the shock, Nick said he wanted to transfer someplace, so we looked at a lot of schools. Bowling Green State University accepted him into the business school and that was the spring of 1997.

SUE: The university was very close to our home, yet he would live there. It was a good choice because he had a hard time leaving our home and his younger brothers, and his heart was still really at St Francis – and so we being young parents thought, well, you need to go away to school; that's what you need to do. We probably should have kept him a little closer to home, even though it was only a couple of hours away – just because he needed that. So, when he went to Bowling Green, he was close enough that he could come home – just a 30-minute drive. In fact, he was able to assist in coaching with his former football coach at St Francis and his brothers were on the team, so it was great because all three of them were together again and he loved it.

TIM: However, a very key point is that, although we have these expectations for our children, we tried not to put on a lot of pressure, but there was just enough. So, in March of 1997, he's going to Bowling Green. We think all was well, but he apparently came home and I think – I don't know if it was Tim and Joe [Nick's brothers], but one of them came into our bedroom and he said: 'Nick tried to take his life.' And we were totally like 'No, what?'

Nick came home and basically said he couldn't do it because he wouldn't want to hurt us. So, we knew enough to know that he needed help.

SUE: From there, we took him to the hospital, and he was evaluated, and he was admitted.

TIM: And here's another mistake that I made, but remember we're not sure about all this. I'll never forget it. The following week my job took me to Mexico. We said either I stay back to be home, or I go to Mexico to try to make it normal. Well, if I had it over to do, I would have not gone to Mexico. So, Sue was kind of left with holding the bag at the hospital, which was a very unfortunate experience.

SUE: In some respects, a lot of things have changed since the nineties, as far as mental health treatment: there's new medications, there's more recognition. We talk about suicide; we talk about mental health more than we ever did back in the nineties. But back then, it was just one of those things we didn't talk about. We didn't know that much about it, particularly with adolescents. I call him an adolescent, but he was actually a young adult. He was 20. Anyway, things have changed a lot since then, thankfully, but there are still some things that haven't.

TIM: There were two things at that time that happened at the hospital. Firstly, he was in with a group of adults. Some of them were drug addicts. They were adults talking about how you could take your own life. I mean, he was a 20-year-old young guy and he's getting this feedback. I have to admit, I still thought Nick had got it together and we think we're going to get through this. Okay, so there were some mistakes made by us, but back then in America there was only 6 million dollars appropriated by Congress for mental health research. Today that has changed.

SUE: We learned a lot of what was going on about Nick not directly from him, but through this friend that I had mentioned earlier that he was close to. He told us that Nick was in a support group at the hospital, and he was with adults, and they basically told him: 'Hey, if you really want to be successful, you get a gun and do it that way.' We didn't find this out until after the fact. We're not gun owners. We've never had a gun. That doesn't mean that we're opposed to people having guns, but it wasn't in our language or our discussions.

TIM: Nick had a psychologist counsellor and was on several medications. That was the second thing. If you do research, you get on a couple of these different medications and they can create suicidal thoughts.

SUE: This was long before black box warnings [a safety warning given to drugs] came about on these medications, because they were new. The SSRIs [selective serotonin reuptake inhibitors], which are a lot of the antidepressants that are popular today, we now know can potentiate suicidal ideation, and I don't speak as an expert on that, although I do have some medical background. But we know that now; we did not know that back in the nineties.

* * *

SUE: How do you control a young adult? You want them to be independent. You want them to make their own decisions. You can't keep them in a bubble. You can monitor some things but, you know, we wanted things to be as normal for him as possible. And in fact, when he was discharged from the hospital, we wanted him to go back to school. We wanted him to get back into his lifestyle, because we felt that that was good for him.

TIM: What haunts me is I wish we would have had him stay at home and go to the University of Toledo, but because Bowling Green was only 30 minutes away I felt like things were getting better. Nick was a very bright guy, and I remember sitting on the bench in front of our house, and we were talking and then he says, 'This is not quality of life for me.' And I said, 'Nick, we're going to beat this thing. We are going to beat it.' So, I guess, from my standpoint, maybe I wasn't accepting it.

Nick, besides being a really good student at Bowling Green, was an assistant coach at St Francis, which is where he excelled. His two brothers, Tim, who's a doctor today and Joe, who's a Penn State NFL player, were on that team. And to me it was like, are you kidding me? I mean, that's where I went to school. That's where I played ball. And it was like, we're there, we're making it. In the meantime, he's on meds, he's getting counselling, and the coaches were super. They were together.

* * *

TIM: Probably another big mistake we made is we kept it confidential. We thought, we're not going to tell our family because we don't want to spook them. And again, mental health was still one of those stigma things.

SUE: I think that was something that we wish we would've done a little differently. We did discuss his condition with Tim's sister because Tim and I and the other two boys, who were still in high school, went on a spring break trip and Nick was going to stay back because he was not on break from university. So, we said we need somebody to kind of watch out and make sure everything's okay. So, we did tell Tim's sister, but we did not – and we have a very large family – discuss it with anyone else.

TIM: So, there were some ups and downs during that time. And his coach used to call us. He'd say, 'Well, you know, we see some things with Nick; he's still going through it.' Then it was October 10th, 1997. I'll never forget it. I was in my office. A receptionist came running and said, 'You have an emergency phone call.' I'm thinking, 'Oh my God.' So, I got on the phone, and it was his friend, and he said, 'Nick's in big trouble. He's out by the high school. He's in a daze. He's spaced out.' I said,

'I'll be there.' So, I get in my car. I zoomed over and Nick was walking around. It was like, this is another nightmare. So finally, the call to the rescue squad got the police, but he would not go inside, and he said, 'You're violating my rights.' So, he finally goes in, they take him to the hospital, and I called Sue, and I'm thinking this is bad, but you know what – we're going to get through it.

SUE: Nick was in the emergency room, and he was having some issues, and he got up and got out of the emergency room and ran out of the hospital. We were sitting out in the waiting room, and we heard this commotion, and we went back to see that he was gone. And I said to the young nurse, 'How could this happen?' She goes, 'Well, I have sicker patients to attend to.' I'm like, 'How sick do you have to be?' Now, remember, this was back many years ago when things weren't as they are today, but it just tore my heart out, especially because I'm a nurse. He was very sick, but it was a mental health sickness that people didn't quite understand like they do a heart attack or whatever.

* * *

TIM: So, we carry on and he gets back to coaching, he's still going to school, and the coaches are still working with us, and there was a soccer game that our son Tim was in. It was a district final, St Francis versus St John's, which is a very big rivalry. We never beat them in soccer but this time we did, and because the stadium wasn't far from Bowling Green, Nick was able to come and watch it.

SUE: It was cold, and I recall he had just a thin white jacket on, and I said to him, 'Nick, aren't you cold?' It's cold in October in Ohio. And no, he said he was fine, but he didn't look fine. He looked drawn; he looked tired. And so, we beat St John's. I mean, it was a huge game, and Nick, who was six foot, six foot one and 215 pounds, runs out onto the field, and tackles Tim and he goes down. Boom. We were all just so excited.

Nick was home for the weekend and he had asked if we could have turkey, so I cooked a nice dinner, and we were just a normal family. It was just a very lovely, lovely weekend.

TIM: Then he had to go back to school, which was a short drive, and he called later on Sunday evening – this is October 26th – and he said he left his wallet at our house, and we said no problem; he could come and get it.

On Monday, October 27th, Sue had gone to work, and I had to drive to a small town in Indiana for work and I'm meeting with managers and that, and I said, 'I gotta get my voicemail.' Well, on that voicemail was Nick, and he said, 'Dad, I'm really sorry. I can't take it any more. I'm leaving.' 'This is it,' I thought. 'Oh my God.' I mean, it was even worse than a nightmare. So, I called Sue. I said, 'Sue, we got a terrible problem.' So, Tim and Nick's friend, they try to go and find him. Sue and I drove most of the evening trying to find him.

SUE: In October, it starts getting dark very early in Ohio and so we didn't know where we were going. We didn't know where he was. We were searching. My family did have a lake house about an hour and a half away and I said, 'Let's just take a drive up there.' So, we did because he had gone there a couple of times by himself. We went up there. We couldn't see any evidence that he had been there but there was a strange box on the porch. Now the lake house was closed for the winter, and there was this long empty box on the front porch and that was unusual because everything had been closed down, but I guess we didn't think too much of it. So, we left and came home.

TIM: However, the neighbour at the lake house had called Sue's dad and said he had heard some pops: boom, boom, boom, boom. We were totally wiped out, totally exhausted, didn't know what to think, but personally I felt like we were gonna find him alive, quite frankly.

SUE: And of course, my dad was upset. Nick had apparently gone over and talked to the neighbour and asked him if he had a key to get into the lake house. And the neighbour then realised there was something not quite right and called my father and my father called me. And that is when I told him that we had been dealing with Nick's illness and my father then became quite concerned. I tried to explain to him that we didn't know what was happening, but we knew something was not good.

TIM: So, from there, we went home, and being strong people with faith, praying our guts out, having people all over the place – a good friend of mine who's a minister in Toledo, we said, 'Please get him on the prayer list' – and things are ticking, ticking, ticking…

Now it's October 28th. Sue and I just said, 'We don't know where this is going but I think we're headed into a danger zone.' Then I think it was about four o'clock in the morning, we heard a knock on the door. I opened it up and it was the police. And we're in a state of shock. We still didn't know what was going on. The police officer looked at me and he said, 'You need to call a detective.' And they were in Ann Arbor, Michigan. And I called, and it was a female detective, and she said, 'I'm very sorry for your loss.'

Now, at that point, and I still get chills thinking about it, it's like, what's happening here? Is this a movie? And I looked at Sue, and Sue looked at me and somehow she kept it together.

SUE: Ann Arbor was about an hour-and-20-minute drive from the lake house. So, we were kind of in the right location – close. We realised later what the long box was on the front porch: it was the box for a gun, a rifle. And the pops that the neighbour had heard, apparently our son had been shooting the gun there, but that is not where they found him. And yes, he did take his life using a gun and he was under the influence of alcohol and medication.

TIM: The psychologist we had talked to, when he took off, had thought that the medication was going to run its course, that he was going to be tired, and he'd fall asleep somewhere. That's what we hoped might happen.

From there, there are really no words. I mean, you can call it a nightmare, but there are no words. And when we start calling our family, they just exploded with grief. It was the worst. Terrible. No words to describe that particular day. And I think we were in such shock that the adrenaline was flowing and that we had to start to look at this now as a process, you know, get ready for a funeral to bury our son.

SUE: As we had not really discussed his illness with our family, they were totally in shock because they had no idea that there was anything like this going on. And maybe that was a mistake. Maybe we should have been a little more open, looking back. I think it takes a village – I hate to use an idiom – but it does take more than just yourself. It's the community and the people you know who want to be there and help you. It's not something to be ashamed of.

TIM: In the community, our family is big in Northwest Ohio. We've got lawyers, we've got doctors, we've got athletes. I mean, Nick was one of the best athletes in the Toledo area. And when that hit the community, they were totally in shock. I don't even know if you can call it shock. Here's this all-American young man and he's gone, by suicide, which at that time, again, nobody talked about.

I mean, we could go on and on and on about the dynamics, the two dynamics that stick in my mind. One, it was Halloween the Friday of that week, and we were playing St John's again, two of the best teams in Northwest Ohio, for the city championship and to go into the playoffs in football, and the coach came to us and said, 'Should we call it off?' and we said, 'No.' And we talked to Tim and Joe, and they said, 'Nick would want to play.' The players from St John's and the coach – who was a good friend of Nick's – came to the funeral home. And all that week we were thinking that this just can't be happening. So, we beat St John's.

And then, there's the funeral on November 1st, my mom's birthday. There were a thousand people in the church – six or seven Oblates were saying the mass again. We're still in shock. Our adrenaline is going; you're still in disbelief. And I think, sometimes as humans we think we're in control. Well, we're not in control. And even though you have an all-American young man, you know what? That has nothing to do with it. You know, even with great accomplishments, it's about the health of your child.

SUE: So, I guess the moral of our story is that suicide can affect anyone. It doesn't have to be someone who's down on their luck. It can be someone who's at the pinnacle. It's just a mental health condition and, unfortunately, we lost our son.

***

TIM: When we lost him, we went to the psychiatrist. The first thing I said was that I didn't know you could die from depression or mental health.

SUE: We thought Nick would get better. We tried to keep life as normal as possible.

Tᴜᴍ: We learned a lot after he passed, because a lot of people came and told us things that we were not aware of. I remember talking to one of his professors, who again said he was a brilliant student, and I said, 'Professor, I thought we were going to beat this thing,' and he said, 'I don't know if you ever beat it,' and that sticks in my mind.

Sᴜᴇ: We've learned a lot, but we still have a lot to learn. Things have changed and I'm not so sure they've changed for the better. Maybe the one thing that's improved is that we're not afraid to talk about it any more. It's out in the open. Mental illness is nothing to be ashamed of. If there are times in your life when sometimes things don't go the way you want them to, it's okay to talk to people about it. Don't feel that you have to keep it to yourself.

Tɪᴍ: Nick's friends came back and told us that they knew he was struggling and that he talked about not wanting to be around any more. And I said, 'Why didn't you tell us that?' But back then, you just didn't do it. You don't go to the parents and say, you know, that something is difficult.

* * *

Tɪᴍ: So, in 2018, we decided to write a book. We felt we were old enough then to deal with it. We wanted our five grandkids to know who Uncle Nick was and here we are 27 years later, and he's still making an impact, especially with his scholarship at St Francis.

SUE: Once we began writing, it flowed very quickly and it's a short read. It's not a long book. It tells the story that no one's immune to tragedy. It tells the story of how we survived the grief and how we worked through the grief.

TIM: The book is called *The Penn State Walk-On* and it tells Nick's story but also the story of our youngest son, his brother Joe, who was a tremendous athlete, at track and football, big guy, you know, like 6'4", 290 pounds. Nick was his mentor and coach, and he said to Joe, 'Whatever you do, you play division-one football or forget it.' Joe had been recruited by some of the big schools such as Ohio State and Yale, but he ended up playing for Penn State, a football powerhouse and one of the top universities in the U.S. He also had an Ivy League School, Penn University, recruit him for track and field. The book gets into how he became this walk-on [a walk-on in college football is a player who joins a team without receiving an athletic scholarship or being recruited], 18 years old with the number-two team – in some cases, number-one team – in the country. So, the book talks about how, all of a sudden, we go from this hell to the light beginning to shine. It was a great distraction.

* * *

TIM: Nick's loss affected our physical and mental health, you know, losing weight, just getting up in the morning, and we had to watch ourselves because you can go down the tubes very quickly if you don't take care of yourself.

SUE: Tim and I both went back to work very quickly, and it wasn't because we were trying to turn it off. We were trying to get back to some sense of normalcy if we could. But there's a lot of people that can't do that. And you know what? You have to accept people where they're at.

We did attend some grief counselling. I went a little longer than the boys and Tim did. We went to some support groups and still maybe, once in a while, we'll attend a support group. I think you have to talk about your feelings. The fortunate thing for Tim and I is our relationship allows us to talk. Sometimes marriages don't survive the loss of a child for whatever reason. And we do have faith, which has helped us tremendously. Communication is really important, so don't be afraid to talk to other folks. If you have to get help from medical professionals, then that's what you need to do. You can't bottle it up. Grief is something you can't run away from. You might think, oh, I'll go on a vacation and things will get better. No, it goes with you. You have to go through the various stages and deal with it. And, you know, at some point you'll stop asking the question, why did this happen? That was something that a very wise person told us, that you'll keep asking that question and eventually you won't ask it any more. You have to learn to accept it.

People would come to me and say, I don't know how you get through this. I would say, 'You don't really want to know, cause which of your children would you give up?' You know? But we learned that we were not alone. There are people that you can talk to, other people that have gone through this: wiser souls, maybe. I think that was our message and our rationale for writing the book – to let people know that you can survive.

One thing we say in the book is that we were given quite a blessing, actually. Joe was the first true freshman walk-on to start for Penn State and his start was almost two years to the day of Nick's death. It was like someone was up there or wherever helping us because we were grieving tremendously, and this was kind of the epitome. We're a big football family. The boys were just really into it. We were into it as a family, and this was an unheard-of kind of thing that happened. It was so unbelievable. There were messages along the way, and we really felt that that was our faith helping us as well.

TIM: Football in the United States is like a religion. The fact that two years later, we had this 18-year-old young guy hitting national news, *USA Today*, *New York Times*, *ABC News*, and it was kind of like it was a gift from God. So, it was a distraction for those next four years. And when Joe made the NFL, it was just like a movie and that's why we say that the light begins shining. When we talk to people, they say that when they read the first chapters of the book and what we went through, many would cry and then the light begins shining.

SUE: We're human beings and we need to accept one another, and we need to understand that at some point in our lives we may suffer from depression and that's part of the human condition. Grief is a very difficult thing. If you're human, you're going to experience grief at some point in time.

Communicating with each other, don't be afraid to talk about it. Don't be afraid. If you hear something, if you believe something's going on, share your thoughts and your feelings.

I think, particularly as parents, if you see something off with a child, maybe it's going to turn out to be nothing, but alert the people that need to know.

TIM: When you go through something like this, you feel like you've lost your hope, which is a terrible feeling. You're in your own world. When you're going through it with a child, or an adult, with mental health problems, you start to lose hope. You've got to keep the hope. Whether you have faith or not, you need something to hang on to. You could just hide your head in the sand and say, 'That's the way it goes.' As we know, life is fragile, and it can change in a second.

We miss Nick every day; there's a missing piece. Death of your child, by suicide or any reason, is not the order that it's supposed to be.

SUE: I don't think men should feel that it's a weakness to talk about mental illness. It isn't a weakness. It's a human condition.

....

Tim and Sue are the authors of *The Penn State Walk-On: Overcoming the Pain and Legacy of Suicide Through Football, Faith, and Family.*

JEFF

EVERYONE NEEDS A BIG, HAIRY-ARSED, AUDACIOUS GOAL

'I used to value small, trivial things. Now I can see what really has value: friendship and family. Sounds corny, but it's true. A beautiful garden, good company, a good bottle of wine. I always drink the best bottle of wine in the rack now. That's a change. I don't save anything for a rainy day. It's today and I'm happy with that.'

I guess I was a little unusual in as much as I knew that I was depressed from about ten or eleven years old. I didn't know the word for it then, but it was something that I felt intensely – that blackness, that hollowness – that none of my contemporaries ever seemed to even understand. I couldn't talk to anybody about it, although I did speak to a teacher at the time who said, 'Oh, you're depressed.' And that's the first time I ever heard the word, and I never really thought any more about it, but of course it was something that revisited me every year with alarming regularity and varying degrees of severity throughout my life. And like Winston Churchill, I call it the black dog; and when the black dog has you, what you need to know is how to respond and recognise the symptoms, and ideally before you get too down.

That's lesson number one I learned. Prevention is a lot better than cure, so avoiding getting depressed in the first place is a much better way to do it. Later in my life, it was a seasonal thing – the shortening days, gloomy weather certainly was a factor. But when I was young, I think it was a symptom of living in a chaotic household. Domestic violence was a factor, and I had a pretty traumatic time, so being depressed around ten years old, it's not really that surprising, to be absolutely honest with you.

I struggled with the depression and just tried to get through it the best I could, I guess like many guys do. I was in my early thirties when I was first medicated and took antidepressants for the first time, and I felt it was quite liberating that I could actually say that I was depressed out loud. My wife knew that I was a sufferer but nobody else really did. I went to see the GP and he did all kinds of tests – looked in my eyes and checked my blood pressure. He could tell from the instant I walked through the door that I was depressed, but he needed to be able to say, 'Well, we've ruled everything else out,' which I was very grateful for.

I took the tablets for several months through one winter and got into the spring, but they did have a rather alarming side effect in that my weight ballooned because they have a big impact on your appetite, particularly for sweet things. And having a bit of a sweet tooth anyway, I wasn't sure whether the juice was worth the squeeze, but it was – even though my weight went up.

I was quite a keen cyclist at the time, and I found that if I exercised pretty vigorously then things didn't seem to get quite so bad or quite as often, and that was the first real inkling that exercise and being outside might help me avoid going down and limit the duration of being there. It wasn't until I was older that I really followed that idea to its ultimate conclusion.

When I was working, one of the things that I did notice, although I don't know whether I was ever diagnosed with this, was certainly an element of being bipolar. I used to talk about, 'I'm really fizzing. I'm really doing well. I'm doing great right now,' but then I also realised the inevitable aftermath of being up is you're going to be down.

I had a conversation with a boss many years ago about this kind of bipolar character. Sometimes you feel *so* good. You can do anything. You're Superman. And he said, 'Is the down worth the up?' And I never really thought of it quite like that. But I don't think I would be able to say, 'No, it's not,' because you do feel great. You feel like you can accomplish anything. You're super confident, but you know what's going to happen. It's like the hamster in the wheel. Things just get faster and faster and faster and faster and faster. And eventually it goes *bang*, and then you're in bed, and you can't face the world for three days and you're scared to go outside, or you're scared to go into a crowded place. All of a sudden, you're a completely different person, and yet, just a few days ago, you were Superman and now you're frightened to go into the café at Marks and Spencer's – the difference is just absolutely amazing but absolutely true.

I used to say to my wife when I was a little bit more informed, 'I need to be careful now, I'm swerving.' I'd just feel that little bit of anxiety and I had learned to recognise it as a symptom. You need to be good to yourself at that point, otherwise it's not going to end well. I think the older you get, the more practice you get at it, and the better you become at it.

The antidepressant, called Prothiaden, worked for me. All it seemed to do to me was make me sleep. One of the things about being depressed is you can sleep but never be rested. And when you're anxious you barely sleep at all, and so having something that is just like a chemical hammer that makes you go to sleep is a very useful thing to have. It's almost like it brings you to a dead stop.

So, I was just living season to season, year to year. A little bit manic, a little bit hyper in the summer, and then I'd get to the winter and I would be dreading that blackness that would envelop me and take over my life. And then you just become small, you just become nothing, you just disappear into nothingness. It's horrible; it's the worst thing in the world for me.

***

I had a pretty good job, and I had a good employer, and there was a nice, informed HR manager and I got on very well with her. One day, it was in September and I knew the winter was coming and I was expecting it to be just like it always was – to go down and to struggle up to Christmas and then limp through Christmas and then get into the real hard slog of January and February and then eventually come out of it. That's what I was prepared for. And I went to see her, and I told her what happens to me and that I hate it. And she said that she could see that I was different and reclusive at certain times and very outgoing at others. So, she suggested that I start working with a psychologist to try and make me the best version of me that I could be – I know this sounds kind of cheesy and soundbitey, but it's true – and to do this they shine light in your dark little corners.

She was a very tough lady. There was nothing wishy-washy about her. She would put her head on one side, and she'd hold her chin meditatively and she'd let me spout on and then she'd say, 'Bullshit. Now what do you really think?' She had no time for anything other than the truth. And I loved her. I absolutely loved her.

This is where we examined a lot of the things that had happened to me as a kid and a lot of those experiences have always been with me. Children from violent and complicated family backgrounds have a thing called hypervigilance, where you know a bad situation is likely to kick off at any moment, and you are hypervigilant to it and always trying to head it off. And I think I kept on doing that. I kept on being hypervigilant throughout the whole of my life. We talked a lot about that, about how that had come about, and about being in a house with a narcissistic bully, a self-centred idiot, for a father.

If you're going to do the talking cure, you've got to fess up. There's no good keeping anything back. You've got to put it out there. I did, and I got a tremendous amount from working with this psychologist.

She revisited the exercise thing and so I started a really rigorous fitness regime. I started running. I had never been a runner, but I started running. I got back on my bike and started cycling, but running was the main thing. And all of a sudden, it was like throwing a light switch. I used to dread the dark, cold, grey, windy, wet, rubbish days of January, and now, well, what better day is there to go for a ten-mile run than today, because what else are you going to do with it? And I'd go out in the morning and run through the cold, through the wet, and then I'd come back at lunchtime and I'd have a buzz, an endorphin high. If they'd just bought me a pair of running shoes instead of the drugs, I could have been there ten years earlier! It really was a massive moment and so I kept on running from that stage, right up until just a few years ago. I'm 64 now, so I probably ran until I was about 62, and then I just transferred to the bike.

* * *

One of the things that the psychologist said to me was, 'I want you to think about that ambition that you've got that you daren't tell anybody about. Something that you have always wanted to do but you daren't tell anybody because they might laugh at you.' She called it the 'big, hairy-arsed, audacious goal.'

She said, 'What we need to do is to give you the confidence to be able to go after it, because there's no point having a goal unless you're going to actually pursue it.'

So, I thought about it, and I came up with two. The first one was that I'd always wanted to play a slide guitar solo in a blues band. And she said, 'Well, why don't you?' She was very pragmatic and said that I needed to learn to play slide guitar and then find a blues band and join it.

It was only two years later and I was standing on stage, in a pub in Oxford, playing a slide guitar solo in a blues band. Two years. I mean, I worked bloody hard at it. It took a lot of commitment, but I did it. And I've been a musician ever since. And I was never really a musician before and now I'm a musician and I'm a guitar player.

That then gave me something that was for me. It wasn't work and it wasn't looking after the kids. It was music. It was a hobby that was for me; that the family can either support or not support; that they can either like or not like. I think it's a big thing for men in their middle years. Sometimes you've been pushed into a corner. You've given up things you like to do – like trains or, I don't know, collecting plant pots – and you need to say, 'Well, this is what I do. This is me. This is what I need.'

I think younger generations are better at it, but my generation is very bad at it. We couldn't wait to give up our hobbies and become old. Everybody is beige and old and plays a bit of golf and goes to the same hotel on a holiday every year.

Learning to play the guitar and play in a band was something that *I* wanted to do. I think it's very easy to feel, when you get into your forties, that you're putting on a few pounds, you're losing your hair, and you've got to have that last hurrah, I guess. Maybe that's what I was doing, but I felt it very strongly. I was very keen to do it, and I was successful at it.

My other 'big, hairy-arsed, audacious goal' was inspired by a book I read by a British lady called Josie Dew, called *Travels in a Strange State*, and it was about this adventurous, twentysomething young woman who packed her bike up, got on a plane to America, and cycled across America. She went from Los Angeles right up to Northern Canada and it was a truly astonishing journey. I can remember thinking, 'You can ride a bicycle across a continent?' It just never even occurred to me that you could do that.

It had a certain perfection to it. It's a physical challenge. It's not that expensive, except in time. It's adventurous and it's admirable. It's a great story to tell in the pub. It's just a great thing to say you've done. So, I read the book and – bearing in mind, at the time, I had children who were four and six – there was no way I was getting on a bike and riding across America anytime soon. But that ambition and that desire never left me. Then when I was coming towards the end of my time at work, it resurfaced and, interestingly, I didn't need to read the book again – the idea was just always there.

I was a manager. I'm an organised guy. I can organise things. I started doing some reading around and contacted a few people who had done this kind of thing before. I bought some gear, did a bit of training, and when I did eventually finish work on the 28th of February 2014, four weeks later I flew to St Augustine in Florida, and I rode my bike to San Diego,

California, all the way across three and a half thousand miles. And it was fantastic. Absolutely fantastic. And it's the strangest thing now because it feels like it happened to someone else.

As a goal goes, it was ideal, because it was all-consuming. I was coming to the end of my working life and it's really easy to kind of miss the person that you were at work. You get used to being somebody at work and people behave differently towards you. They just do; it's just human nature. One thing I can tell you is that the day you retire, 24 hours later, nobody cares what you used to do. You have got a shelf life and as soon as it's over nobody cares what you used to do. It's brilliant to see people trying to hang on to it. I find it so funny. I want to put my arm around them and say, 'Give it up, mate. You're not the bank manager any more.' You're just an old man in a beige suit unless you choose not to be. And that's what it's about really.

In your thirties and forties, find your thing, hold on to your thing, despite what pressures you're under, like doing the school run or giving up your nights playing poker or whatever it is; it doesn't matter – hang on to it, hold on to it firmly. Then later on in life, don't have hobbies, have passions, have something that makes you wake up in the morning and say, 'I've got to go and do that,' because if it's just 'yeah, yeah, yeah' it's not going to stick; and when you do finish work, there's a lot of time to fill, and guys are not any good at doing that.

* * *

Having achieved two big goals, my mental health was more manageable, more in control, and with my exercise regime, which I started in my early forties until my sixties, I never had another episode of being truly depressed. I had off days. We all have off days, but I mean something that lasts a substantial period of time, a two-week or three-week period of seriously being off.

So, I'm in my early sixties, I would say fat and happy, but I wasn't fat, because I was fit. I was cycling. I wasn't overweight. I didn't smoke. I had a good diet, although I was a little bit too keen on the biscuits, a bit too much sugar; but because you're burning calories on the bike, I didn't think it mattered. Or so I thought.

And then two years ago, I was just at home playing with my grandson, and all of a sudden I couldn't see out of one of my eyes and my left arm felt like it wasn't attached to me. And I thought, 'This is not good.' I didn't quite know what to do and I ended up phoning NHS 111, and I got this lovely lady on the phone. She said, 'The symptoms you're describing require immediate hospitalisation. There is an ambulance on its way to you.' And literally, as she said those words, the front doorbell rang and there's an ambulance there! It all just kind of swirled and took on a life of its own. I'm there playing with my grandson one minute and the next I'm in an ambulance on the way to the hospital.

I ended up being diagnosed with a TIA, a transient ischemic attack, or a mini stroke. I had an MRI scan, and they found a blocked carotid artery in my neck. I always remember what the stroke doctor told me. He said, 'Patients with your presentation will progress to a life-threatening, often fatal stroke within a very few weeks. So, we'd like to get you in quite soon.' *Quite soon.* I loved the understatement.

I was pretty much straight in within a couple of days, and they took the plaque out of my neck, and I saw it and it was quite a horrible-looking thing. And the surgeon said, 'Oh yeah, that was going to have a bad outcome for you and it absolutely had to be done.' I'm insanely grateful to the skill of the surgeon, but mainly to the young junior doctor who, when I was getting moved from pillar to post in A&E, and I'd been there all day and wanted to go home – typical old man – said, 'I think you've had a TIA, and I'm going to refer you to the stroke team.' And had I not seen her, I would've gone home, and I would have slipped through the net, through my own stupidity. I owe her my life and the quality of life that I have now; and if I ever met her again, I would thank her.

The stroke was a shock. I don't have the words to describe how great a shock it was and the free fall that I went into pretty much immediately. It was the most horrible experience, because of course I was very depressed again.

Following the operation, I was admitted to the ward overnight, given pain relief, then the next day shown the front door: 'Out you go, thank you very much, and have a load of tablets to take for the rest of your days.' And that's pretty much what happened. I'd had this massive shock, this massive change happened, and I just felt like a shadow. I didn't feel like I was real. I certainly didn't feel like me. I'm used to getting on with it: 'We'll have some fun...' That's my way, and instead I'd just sit quietly for hours. I went out with some friends and I just sat there. I couldn't stay. I had to leave; it was just too much. And it took me a while to work out that I was grieving the loss of who I'd been. That took a great deal of coming to terms with, and then it took a long time to get my medications right. I didn't cope very well with one of the drugs they gave me, and we got that changed.

And then the stage I went through next was quite simply anger. I was as mad as hell that this had happened to me and not to the guy who eats pizza for breakfast, drinks beer, and smokes 40 cigarettes a day. He didn't have the stroke – I had the stroke. And that just seemed fundamentally unfair. It's ridiculous, but that's how I felt. I was angry at cycling that it hadn't protected me. I felt like a fool for having believed that this won't happen to me; this will happen to people who don't look after themselves; this will happen to people who abuse their bodies; this will happen to someone else; and yet it happened to me, and I had to suck that up, and it took me two years before I could say I was over it and could see it in perspective.

The interesting thing is that I did the usual thing, you know, came out of hospital, thought 'I'll give this two weeks and then I'll be back on my bike'. Two weeks later and I was like a jelly. I had unrealistic expectations of a return to normal life and that I wasn't going to be beaten by it and, of course, I was just flattened by it. And a fortnight became a month, and a month became three months.

I didn't do any work in my garden. My garden is very important to me. I just didn't engage at all. The only place I felt safe was in bed, in the shower, or playing my guitar. Every other time, every other second of the day, hypervigilance was back, that anxiety was back, and it was just the most horrible time, and it went on, and on, and on. I had some beautiful gestures; people did some beautiful things for me to try and bring me back into the world – and I just couldn't. I had to take my own time.

One of the symptoms that I had, which confused the hell out of me, even a month post-operative, was that I was so tired. I would sleep until ten in the morning, then I'd mooch around until two. I'd go back to bed for two or three hours, get up at five, and I'd be back in bed by ten that evening and that just wasn't like me. I didn't know what was going on. I couldn't get any sense out of the GP at all – couldn't get to even speak to him. So, I phoned the Stroke Association, and they were absolutely fantastic. This young woman I spoke to said, 'Oh yeah, of course. Fatigue's the most common side effect of having a stroke. Everybody's exhausted. It lasts about six months, love. Don't worry about it; everybody goes through it.' And I thought, 'Why didn't anybody tell me? It would have been so much easier!'

They put me in touch with a stroke survivor, and he was a fantastic guy, just what I needed. He'd had a much harder time than I had and yet he was funny, engaging, irreverent, and supportive. He was also well informed and pragmatic, and he'd say things like, 'Don't be in a rush, buddy, just, you know, pick one thing in a day that's better.' And he said, 'One thing I tried to do was kind of *force* recovery, and what I came to realise was that each day I was better, but I was only one per cent better, or maybe half a per cent better, but you're better and you've got to accept that.' It's at a very, very slow rate. Now, he had to learn to talk again, had to learn to walk again. I had nothing but admiration for that man. All I had to do was start feeling like me again and get my energy back.

But to get back to being me took two years and I was very depressed for a long, long time. It was only very gradually that I came back. And then I came through a couple of winters, and I came into spring and then just decided to get back on the bike again, start cycling again, and that helped. Then the more recovery I made, the better I felt, and it's just been a continuous, gradual, slow improvement, not a revolution like I somewhat stupidly expected it to be.

So today, I'm back with all that entails. I'm much more humble than I was. I'm a much better listener. My wife says I'm kinder, which I quite like and made me cry. I've got time for things that I didn't have time for before. The peculiar thing is that I can make it into a positive experience because I used to think I was going to live forever. We all do. I mean, it's stupid when you say it, but our behaviour says we think we're going to live forever, because we don't prepare for old age. We don't prepare for serious illness or anything like that – we just saunter on like we're going to go on forever.

We live in houses that are too big, way too old. We don't dispose of things to people who can actually use them; we just hoard them. Stupid. So, I was going to live forever. And then this came along and smacked me on the side of the head and said, 'Hey, big shot, you know what, you're not.' And I very nearly didn't. I very nearly shuffled off this mortal coil. And if you can't get that lesson and it changes you in a big way, well, if that's the case, I'd quite like to speak to that person just to see what on earth is going on in their head. For me, it has been completely life-changing.

I used to value small, trivial things. Now I can see what really has value: friendship and family. Sounds corny, but it's true. A beautiful garden, good company, a good bottle of wine. I always drink the best bottle of wine in the rack now. That's a change. I don't save anything for a rainy day. It's today and I'm happy with that.

NICO
TURNING A LIFE AROUND: FROM ADDICTION AND CHAOS TO A LIFE OF PURPOSE

'Men need support groups, whether they want to admit it or not. Your golf buddy is your support group. Your fishing buddy is your support group. Your pub buddy, your drinking buddy, that's your support group. That's what our community needs. Everybody's got to put their pants on in the same way, regardless of if you're across the pond or over here in America. And so, if you can do it, then someone else can do it.'

Many of the situations that we run into nowadays come from how we thought or how we were trained to think from our younger years. I grew up in a two-parent household here in Albuquerque, New Mexico. Both my mother and father were present in my life, which was great. I also had an extended family around me, so my tíos [uncles], my tías [aunts], and my cousins, and we spent lots of time together. The hub of the family was mainly at my grandmother's, where we would spend all day playing around and having a really enjoyable time.

My formative years were great, but there were problems which stemmed from the situation with my younger sister. She's two years younger than me and, although she was born healthy, during a checkup as a baby one of the doctors messed up and she got really sick. They told my parents that my sister wasn't gonna make it past one year of age, and that threw them into a whirlwind of 'What do we do? We have a son; we have a daughter, and she is not going to live past year one.'

What I learned later was that my grandmother would come to the hospital and take me back to her house to look after me, so from the age of two to six I spent my time on the road back and forth between Albuquerque, New Mexico, and Flagstaff, Arizona, where she lived.

The thought processes that we have with situations and circumstances from our adolescence, even our very formative years – from zero to seven, and then from seven to twelve – have a tremendous impact on how we think and how we view the world as an adult.

Aged 30, when I eventually came to reflect on the root causes of my behaviours and poor choices, I followed a process where I went back in my life, in reverse, to try and find where some of these things started. I reversed back to when I was 29, and asked myself a series of questions: was there anything that made me feel like I was rejected? Was there anything that made me feel like I was missing out? Was there anything that made me feel like I had been taken advantage of? Was there anything that had made me feel like change was scary? And the last one that I asked myself: was there anything that made me have the need to be right all the time? Was there a fear of being wrong?

After age 29, I went back to 28, 27, and I repeated the process all the way back as far as I could remember. I believe the way to open it up is to be honest with yourself and so, when you go searching for the answers, they're going to pop up. And that's how I found out that the issues of rejection and a fear of missing out were constant themes in my life. It was not easy, and it wasn't fun, but it was something that I needed to do in order to mend and heal. I learned that the fear of rejection and missing out manifested in a need to be included. I needed relationships. We all need relationships, but it was a significant need for me, and it was something that I needed to have all the time.

It was in my early teens that my poor choices started to lead to poor behaviours. I found myself as a 'newbie' in a new high school in a new location. I didn't know anybody at the school, so I started hanging out with individuals who would accept me. However, just because somebody accepts you, it doesn't mean you should spend time with them, and I would spend time with individuals who probably weren't the best choices.

When I was 14 years old, I was invited to hang out with individuals who I later found out were gang members. And because they were people who included me, I didn't see a problem with it. I didn't qualify their behaviours. I didn't qualify their actions and ask myself if I wanted to hang out with individuals who conduct themselves in this way – I just saw somebody who wanted to hang out with me. I saw somebody who wanted to accept me.

And then I would do things just to be accepted. I would get out of my own character in order to be accepted. There's a phrase in Spanish that my grandmother used to say to me, '*Dime con quién andas y te diré quién eres*,' and it means 'Show me who you spend your time with, and I'll tell you what kind of person you're going to be.' So, I was spending my time with individuals who were disgruntled against their parents, who were rebellious, who had aggressive tendencies, and who participated in substance use.

To be accepted amongst my peers, substance use was my way in. The aggression was already there. I wrestled from age seven till seventeen, so I knew how to handle myself whenever they would try to rough me up. It wasn't difficult for me to kind of fight back, so I could stand my ground. The rebellious behaviours and the disgruntled emotions towards my familial group – we shared that one. The only place that I didn't fit in was with the substances. I vividly remember the first time that I got high. I had gotten out of school and one of them was like, 'Hey, we'll give you a ride home, so you don't have to catch the bus today.' I was like, 'Cool, I get to hang out with people,' because when I would get home I was the only one there. My mom and dad were out at work and, despite everything, my sister ended up surviving and she was at a different school.

I got in the car, and I knew what cannabis smelled like and they were smoking it. Well, the blunt got passed around the car and came to me and I was faced with the decision – either I participate in the behaviour, or I don't. In that moment, I made the choice to participate in the use of cannabis. I don't want anyone to think that it was a gateway drug and that's what started it. No, it was my choice to break my own character, my own conscience, and what I knew was right or wrong. And that was the gateway there. It was when I broke character. Even at that young adult age, I then started to implement that behaviour over and over again, and it continued from 14 until I was 27 years old.

I started to smoke cannabis, but I found that my friends liked to smoke tobacco too. So, I found a way to get hold of tobacco products, and I'd sell them to these friends to be included, and I found a way to make some extra money. In my head, I didn't have a problem with it, but apparently we began to cause a ruckus at the school. So, the principal talked to the wrestling coach, because I was a part of the wrestling team, and the wrestling coach talked to my parents and told them that this young man probably shouldn't be hanging around with the people that he's hanging around with and if he continues to he's gonna go down the wrong path, and my parents made the decision to take me out of that school and put me in another school.

Well, the town that I grew up in, Albuquerque, where I still live, is very small so just because I moved schools didn't mean that I moved mindset – I didn't move behaviours. I had already found what actions got me accepted amongst my peer group, and at that point it was solidified in my head that those actions allowed me to be included and let me hang out with other groups of people, not just my own group of friends at that time.

Most teenagers want to participate in smoking something, regardless of whether they're emos or jocks – most people are experimenting around that age. And I leveraged that because I could obtain certain substances and sell them. The high that came from the substances was not nearly as high as being included and being accepted, because that was the missing factor for me. When I got it, my brain would release that dopamine because what we need is community. That's one thing I've learned all my journey. We need individuals to stand alongside with. And we need people to stand against, quite honestly. Those people were the ones that didn't participate in the same behaviours as us. And because I could get cannabis, well, 'Nico, can you get anything else?' And I started to explore other opportunities and that escalated, by choice of course, to obtaining cocaine and pills.

I was born in 1990, so I grew up in the early 2000s, and that's when pills started to really take hold here in America. You could get a pill for anything, and they were giving them out for everything, and so no longer did you have to go to the local drug dealer; you could go to someone's mom, someone's dad, and offer to pay them for their pills – you just gave them a couple bucks and I'd then go sell them.

And so that's where the behaviours started to solidify themselves. I think that it was about being able to solidify my place in the world and that made me excited about what I was doing. The 'moral reasoning' was that if my parents didn't have to take care of me and I could take care of myself, then that would help them out. So that was my point. It wasn't so much a legitimate reason, but I was able to identify myself, and having an identity is important.

And then I was able to carve out my place in the world, because we all want to fit in somewhere, and I say that because there might be people reading this right now who have the career that they have because of an identity that was pressed upon them when they were young. They might have a certain standard of living that they don't even care about, but it is an identity that they have become attached to and that's why they're participating in those daily actions and that's what is causing them internal tension. That's causing them to turn to vices, to turn to behaviours, to turn to pornography, to turn to overeating, to turn to whatever it is that they're turning to, because inside they don't really want to live the way that they're living, and when you can be honest with yourself, then you can honestly move forward.

And that's where peace comes from. Yes, my story has resilience. Yes, my story has transformation; but at the end of the day, what I have been searching for my whole life is peace, and the only time that I found peace in my life was when I accepted who I am naturally, who I am at my core. And for me, that's a person who loves to help individuals, but also needs to set a standard. I'm a standard setter and that's where I believe identity comes into play – I attach to that identity more than to the person I was when I was rebelling against my parents when I was 20 years old, which led me to getting detained for armed robbery.

* * *

Because of the amounts of drugs that I was using and the path that I had chosen to take, I got a reputation for doing things that were risky. One day I got a call from one of the guys that I knew, and he said, 'Hey, my buddy is going to be robbing some people. Would you like to participate and get some of the cut?' I had no problem with that, so this guy tells me where to meet him and that me and this individual, who I don't know, are going to go on our own, which again was no big deal. It was just a job to me. So, this individual gets in my car. He says, 'We gotta make two stops and then we're gonna go get these guys.'

As we're driving, we're getting to know each other. We're getting to feel each other out, because it's my first time interacting with this individual. And we go to the apartment that he was at, and he picks up a gun there. We go to this other apartment, and we pick up some drugs, because most of the time we were participating in these behaviours intoxicated.

We end up calling these guys and meeting up with them behind a local grocery store. And I'm sitting in the truck. I got this single-cab vehicle. I'm in the driver's seat. We're playing some music. The cab is full of cigarette smoke and we're both high and you can just feel this heaviness in the space, because we're both at attention, because I met this guy less than an hour ago and now we're about to go commit a crime together.

He tells me, 'I know these young kids – they got a bunch of pills. We're gonna set them up.' And I said, 'All right, cool. You rob them and I'll make sure that we get away.' I told him to make sure to get their cell phones and their wallets. He cocks his gun. We pull up behind this Chrysler sedan and he calls one of the guys and he gets out of his vehicle, which is in front of us.

The individual that I'm with gets out of my car and they meet in between the vehicles. I can see him pull out the gun and put it in this guy's stomach. Well, unfortunately, the guy who we were robbing laughed at him and this individual did not take that well. He grabs him by the back of the head, and he grabs the butt of the gun and slams him in the face with it and I could see teeth go flying from his mouth. I look inside of their vehicle and there's another guy inside the car. Well, the individual that I'm with grabs the drugs, but he forgets to grab the wallets and the phones. The reason why we want to take the wallets and the phones is because, firstly, I wanted their identities in case something cracked off and we needed to take further action and, secondly, I didn't want them to call the police.

The situation escalated at a rate that neither of us were prepared for. Once he got the drugs, he went to the car and pulled out the other guy and took all his drugs too. So, we got all the drugs, but we didn't get any of the stuff that would kind of protect us – the phones and the wallets. He gets back in my vehicle. He still has his gun, and he puts it on his lap, so it's now directed at me.

I accelerate and I make a right down this street, make a left and make another right to try and get out of the area. I get onto this main road so we can go to this park and we can leave my truck there and we won't get caught. As I'm driving down the street, this cop car pulls out behind us and all of a sudden the lights go on and this individual says, 'Outrun them.' I was not outrunning them, because the truck is in my name, and it's registered to my parents' house. Even if I try to outrun the cops, I'm not going to send them over to my parents' house.

So, I pull over. I had been in other situations with the police where I knew how to charismatically get my way out of it, speak to them in certain ways, and deny everything, so I think that if neither of us tell, then we're good to go. But because our relationship was new, there wasn't any trust between us, and as soon as I pulled over he opened up the door and he booked it, and I just watched him take off. In my head, he had just ratted us out and I was pissed because, by running like that, he was essentially telling them that we did something wrong.

The cop pulls out his gun and he's standing behind his car door telling me to put my hands on the roof of my car. They call in another set of police and all of a sudden I have ten police behind my vehicle with assault rifles. I can see the red dots from their lasers inside my truck.

It takes about 15 or 20 minutes for them to approach me, pull me out of the vehicle and then they bring a gentleman out of the cop car and put a spotlight in my face so that I can't see. I know there were only two people in the car we robbed; one of them was missing teeth and must now be on his way to the hospital, so it had to be the other one who now identified me, so I got detained on armed robbery.

I was blessed enough to have a lawyer on hand. My family knew a lawyer and they helped me out in beating the charge. I never got sentenced, never got imprisoned, but I was very lucky in that situation because, without that lawyer, I probably would've gone to prison.

***

That type of event is what got my attention because that's when I learned that the identity that I had was not the identity that I wanted to have. I was pursuing being this individual who could handle situations like that, which wasn't the person I am.

And that's where a lot of the transformation came from. All I was searching for was peace and acceptance. So, I challenge anybody reading this: how are you? What extreme things are you doing where you are putting yourself in risky situations? I know it might be not as risky as the ones that I've experienced, but you are risking something. Are you risking the peace of mind that you have because your conscience isn't clear?

In my community, it's very likely for individuals to get caught up in this behaviour. I would say on average about 70 per cent of individuals will probably conduct themselves in this way. And that's just in my community here in Albuquerque, but I would say it's also the case here in America and anywhere that the gangster lifestyle is promoted as being very attractive. Having this type of anti-traditional route is something that will always be attractive.

Why is it attractive? I believe it's when it is the most attractive option out there. We all want to be somebody who can be admired. If that is defined as an individual who takes charge, an individual who solves problems, an individual who isn't going to be taken advantage of, then why wouldn't you want to be like that? So, on average, my guess would be about 70 per cent of the community gets caught up in some form of this, whereas 30 per cent never even participate.

* * *

I wish I could say the armed robbery charge was rock bottom, but it was not. Unfortunately, that happened when I was only 20 years old. When I was 22, a couple of events happened that compounded the situation.

I grew up around one of those 30 per cent guys. He was one of my good friends and he had a younger brother. It was New Year's Eve, and I partied, I went out with the girl that I was seeing, we had a great time, we partied, we did all those things – drink, smoke, sex, all of it. The next day I get a call like 6 or 7 in the morning, and my buddy is telling me, 'Nico, my brother's gone.' I'm like, 'Well, where'd he go?' He's like, 'My brother's dead.' And again, he's in the 30 per cent. He was a guy that never participated in any of these behaviours. So, I scramble myself together and I go to meet up with him. It turns out his younger brother had gone to a party and taken drugs that were given to him, and he didn't wake up the next day and had just passed away from whatever he ingested.

That stood out to me because, at this point in my life, I was doing probably about four or five 80 milligram OxyContin pills a day, I was smoking weed on a constant, consistent basis and drinking. And to hear that somebody had passed away from an overdose so close to me kind of shocked my brain. But I didn't stop. Because during my twenties, I'd already been through things where I thought, 'Well, if this didn't take me out, then that won't take me out,' and I had that kind of arrogance and cockiness that comes with it.

It was a few months later that I had an eviction notice on my apartment. I wasn't managing my money correctly any more and I found myself sleeping in my vehicle in a Walmart parking lot because I didn't have the wherewithal to see how much my quality of life had deteriorated because of my substance use.

So, those events made me feel like a failure, made me feel rejected, made me feel isolated. And that's when I decided to stop using opiates. The unfortunate part is that I didn't understand that alcohol was a substance as well. I just replaced one with the other. So, from the ages of about 24 to 27, I was excessively drinking and I found myself in the same cycle: being isolated from my family because I wasn't a very nice drunk and being isolated from my friends because I had changed my demeanour so much that they didn't want to be around me. The person that they did like as a friend, I was no longer that individual.

I then started living in a building that only had electricity, mainly because my mom said, 'Here, your grandma left this house. If you want to stay in it you can, but it better not be your coffin.' I realised that I had really been messing up because of the choices that I had been making and because of the people that I had been spending time with. I was not realising the outcomes that I ultimately wanted. There had not been a consistent group that accepted me. I always had to do something to have that acceptance, like it was a quid pro quo. If you do this for me, I'll do this for you. That's what the relationship was. It wasn't true friendship. It wasn't true camaraderie.

* * *

I grew up in a household that believed in religion. For me, because I didn't like authority, I had been anti-religion, anti-authority. I didn't want to be told what to do. But there's going to be somebody you have to listen to, and if it's not going to be the available authorities – your parents in your childhood – then, as you get into your adulthood, the community that you live in provides the authority that you must follow. So, I decided that I was going to explore what this religion really was and to take a spiritual path towards changing my life.

And so, when I was 27, I reached out and I talked to this God that my parents had taught me, and it transformed my life. Nothing about me physically changed, other than no longer having the need and desire for substances. My job didn't change. The work that I was doing didn't change. I still lived in my grandma's abandoned house, but I had the peace that I was always searching for. I had the acceptance, and it filled all the needs that I wanted. There was consistency in something that was greater than me.

I believe that each day we are given is a gift, and so that's where the real transformation came from for me. And in that conversation and transformation, I realised that everything that I had gone through was an opportunity to teach someone else.

I learned that I was the only one that could control my thoughts and my actions. And I began to transform those not at a spiritual level, but at a very practical level. The way I used to think wasn't helpful, so I had to transform every thought that came into my head because, I realised, they were not my thoughts – just passing notifications. By capturing it and either accepting it or rejecting it, I was able to change the way that

I felt; and by changing the way that I felt, I changed the way I chose to take action. I call this TEA: Thoughts, Emotions, Actions. If you can capture and start with the thoughts, then you can change the way that you emotionally feel. And if you change the way you emotionally feel, you can change your actions.

By doing that, I was able to achieve a higher education. I ended up getting a job that paid for my schooling. I was able to write a book. I was able to stop all substances at this point in my life. I can proudly say that I don't drink, I don't smoke, I rarely use caffeine – only when I absolutely need to, because that's a substance to me. Sugar is another substance; artificial sugar is a substance in my world and I'm clean of all those substances. I participate in daily physical activity that helps me stay regulated. It's one of my coping mechanisms. I journal and I read. And those are the ways that I stay healthy; and by implementing those behaviours on a day-to-day basis, that's how I made the change into the individual that I am today.

* * *

In my opinion, you should have three people around you at all times. Somebody who's ahead of you, where you want to be basically. Somebody who's right next to you, going along the same path at the same pace. And then somebody behind you, who's coming up and is usually a mentee that you can share some of your wisdom with.

One of my mentors asked me, 'Nico, what are you an expert in?' And I was like, 'Well, I'm an expert in getting clean.' I knew that drugs and alcohol weren't the out that I needed, but once I got into them it was hard to stop, and I wasn't going to go to rehab. I wasn't going to go to jail. I didn't believe in those modalities for myself. I figured if I could get myself into these positions, then I should be able to get myself out of these positions. And so, when they asked me that question, my immediate answer was, 'I know how to get clean.' And he said, 'Well if you know how to get clean, can you teach it to people?' And so that's where the book came from.

I identified the common theme every time that I got clean, but there also was a gap that I noticed in the realm of recovery and that was that people would talk about what to do when you're in rehab, what to do after you're in rehab, but nobody talked about what to do *before* you even get to those places. And so the book addresses the decision that you have to make before the decision.

Statistically, I'm in the 1 per cent of people who used the amount of drugs that I used and drank the amount that I drank and now can say that I'm where I am as a published author with my own business. I am one of the lucky ones. For me though it's just daily life. It was just surviving another day and doing it in the best way that I can. Because that's one thing that I will say about my life: whatever I'm going to do, I'm going to do it to the best that I can. So, if I'm going to be selling dope, then I'm going to sell dope the best way that I know how to do it. If I'm working just a normal job, cleaning toilets, or taking calls in a call centre, I'm going to be the very best at it. And for me, that's been the biggest driver.

I don't like to look at it as luck because, in my head, the work that I do now is to honour those that can't do it. I do it for the people that I know who've died. I do it for the mothers that I know are struggling right now with loving a son, loving a husband, loving a nephew who is hurting and they're doing everything that they can, and they just can't reach him.

The way that I conduct myself now is what I used to think was hard. And so that's why I do it. As a teenager, I used to think that running around, running amok, causing problems, was hard and that's why I did it. So now for me, the hardest thing to do is to be the best example and serve my community, serve people who are truly seeking to better themselves, because I've learned how to transform myself. I've shot up heroin. I've smoked crack. I've done acid. I've done robberies. I've done breaking and entering. I've been in fights. I've done all of that. But I've also written books. I've also got higher education. So whichever side they want to discuss, I now have the skills to do it.

Men need support groups, whether they want to admit it or not. Your golf buddy is your support group. Your fishing buddy is your support group. Your pub buddy, your drinking buddy, that's your support group. That's what our community needs. Everybody's got to put their pants on in the same way, regardless of if you're across the pond or over here in America. And so, if you can do it, then someone else can do it. You need to be the example. Do better today in creating that example.

....

Nico is the author of *Five Things to Know Before You Get Sober.*

SHAY
RECLAIMING INTIMACY AND TACKLING BEDROOM ANXIETY

'When we're watching porn, it's not like real-life sex – it doesn't happen that way – but our brain doesn't know the difference. Our brain doesn't know that we're watching it through a screen. So, the same chemicals are released in our body as if we were actually with somebody, but it's supercharged.'

There was life before 2018 and then there was life after 2018. Life before 2018 was 12 years in banking. On the surface, everything appeared great in life in terms of a nice house, a nice car, I could buy what I wanted to, could go where I wanted to in the world, all these kinds of things. Everything looked great. But actually, I had a really bad relationship with pornography and with sex, which at the time I thought was all very normal. I thought, well, every guy watches porn, and it's normal to engage in regular hookups. I didn't actually realise the amount of destruction this was causing in my life, and I wasn't going to realise that for another five years or so.

* * *

I would say my porn addiction was generally a daily thing. Sometimes it could be more than once daily. Sometimes it could be less than that. I now understand it is more about the relationship that we have with porn, as opposed to the frequency of watching it, and the patterns that I'm creating in my mind. Am I creating a pattern that says porn is more enjoyable than sex with an actual person?

There are multiple needs that porn meets, so for me I would say that's where the frequency was, but over a long period of time. I think the statistics now are something like, by the age of eight, 80 per cent of boys have watched porn, because it's so accessible. There's no hiding from it. I think I was part of the first generation that had access to smartphones and high-speed internet, so it was there, whatever you wanted to see, for free and immediately accessible. I wouldn't say I was choosing porn over sex, but on reflection I would say it was one of the factors that had started to impact my performance in the bedroom – but at the time I had no idea. All I knew was that I had this sense of frustration with my life, and it wasn't going in the direction that I wanted it to. I noticed that I was pushing people away or feeling quite agitated when it came to conversations with people. It wasn't that porn was the number-one thing – there were other things as well – but it was one of the main factors that were impacting my life. I had this sense of frustration. And then I also started to notice impacts in the bedroom in terms of erection quality and performance.

* * *

Then fast forward to 2018. I decided to quit the corporate world, put on a backpack, and travel the world. The experience just totally changed my life. Anybody that's travelled, you'll know that it is an incredible experience. It opened my mind to taking my life in the direction that I wanted to and realising that I wasn't just this cog in the machine of the corporate world. I could design a future for myself and step out on my own two feet.

So, when I came back, I knew that I didn't want to go back to the corporate world. I wanted to do something for myself, but I had no idea what to do. I just had this voice saying to me, 'Get back out into the world and learn.' So, I started to listen to podcasts and read books. I hadn't read books for years and years, but I started to read mindset and self-development books, and go to seminars. And then I felt this whole expansion of my mind just happened, which then led me to get a coach. And this is the ultimate thing that then led to the trigger being pulled. So it was that step-by-step journey of travelling first, then not knowing what to do, but just knowing I needed to learn more, taking my learning about myself to a whole other level, which led to a coach, and then a conversation happened.

Many people are familiar with Tony Robbins, who's a self-development expert, and he has a set of coaches who work on his models and his principles. I went to a few of his seminars, and I really liked the way that he looked at human psychology and human behaviour. I'd already made a commitment to myself that I wanted to take my life to the next level from what I thought was previously possible, and now I realised there was a whole different life that was possible for me, but I needed some guidance and help to get there.

One of the offers was a coaching package with one of his trained coaches. I had a 12-month package working together with a coach. It wasn't until month 11 that I mentioned anything about sex, hookups, and porn, because I was so embarrassed. I did not know what to say. I didn't want to talk about it. I think, especially as men, we think, 'I just need to figure this out for myself and get it sorted. I don't need to ask for help. I don't need to ask for guidance.' But there are times in our life when we absolutely do need guidance and help, when we don't have the tools or what we have tried hasn't been working. That's when we need external support.

I had got to this point where I was just really frustrated. The businesses that I was trying weren't working. I was questioning myself and it felt like my self-esteem was through the floor, and

I'd never really felt like that before. I was always a confident guy, I'd had a successful career in banking, and I was just thinking, 'What the hell is going on? Why can't I figure this out?'

So, it got to a point where eventually I had a conversation with my coach and she asked me to do this drawing of three circles, and I had to draw the size of the circle to represent the time and energy that I was putting into these three different areas. One was business, one was self-development, and one was relationships.

At this point, I was single and had been for a couple of years. My last relationship had finished, and part of the reason was because of what was going on in the bedroom, and then porn usage escalated and a bad relationship with sex escalated; but when I drew these three circles, I saw the relationship circle was three times the size of the other two circles. And I looked at it, and I thought something's not right here because I'm not in a relationship and it doesn't feel good there's that much time and energy going into that circle.

And that's when it literally felt like the floor just opened up and swallowed me, and I just had this massive slap around the face as I realised that all of this frustration, all of what is going on right now, was linked to porn, hookups, and this whole area of sexual intimacy.

And it was one night in December 2021, I remember the phone call. I remember the room that I was in. And that was the night that I made two commitments. One was to get it sorted for myself because I knew it was a mindset thing – it wasn't a medical thing that was going on. It was mindset, as it is for most men. Then the second commitment was to help other men. Once I'd figured it out for myself, I would then help other men to do the same.

* * *

The needs that porn meets are mainly related to dopamine. When we're watching porn, it's not like real-life sex – it doesn't happen that way – but our brain doesn't know the difference. Our brain doesn't know that we're watching it through a screen. So, the same chemicals are released in our body as if we were actually with somebody, but it's supercharged. As we know, in porn, it's not about the build-up. It cuts straight to the action scene. It's not about stopping or that's enough – it's always more, more, more. We can watch whatever content we want to, immediately, instantly, just like that, so the level of stimulation is unnatural. The level of dopamine that's released in the body is unnatural at this point.

And what happens over time is usually the type of porn that is watched will become a bit more edgy, a bit more extreme, or we'll explore new categories because we're trying to chase the same dopamine high. Just like with drugs. A drug addict doesn't usually start on heroin; they'll start on something softer and then it will build up over time. Same with gambling. It doesn't start with, 'Let's put a hundred grand down in the casino.' It starts with, 'Let's put down a few dollars or a few pounds,' and then we're chasing the high. It's exactly the same thing with porn. Then what happens over time is, when it comes to real-life sex, it's not possible to release the same amount of dopamine. So, we're not able to get hard. We're not able to get as stimulated or turned on in that moment because our mind is used to a whole different level of getting turned on.

The mind is saying, 'This just isn't doing it for me,' whilst the chemicals are still being released – dopamine being the main one – it's just not being released at the same level as when we watch porn, because that's so much more hyper-stimulating. The body's still doing what it should be doing, but it's just doing it at level one instead of level ten when it's with porn.

But there are three other needs that porn is meeting that it's important to be aware of. The first one is that we don't have the fear of rejection. When a guy is alone watching porn, there's no fear of the person walking out of the room. There's no fear of us approaching someone we find attractive and them saying no. So, the fear of rejection is not there.

The second thing is performance anxiety. It doesn't exist when we're watching porn. There is not someone there. We're not thinking, 'I've got to stay hard' or 'What if I'm going to come too quickly?' or 'What if I'm not doing it right?' There's not a sense of that when we're watching porn, because we're alone, safe in our own room. There's nobody else there that we have to cater for, and this leads to the third point: we don't have to worry about whether they are enjoying it. Are they having a good time? Is this what they like or is it something else that I don't know about? We just don't have these kinds of thoughts.

So, those three things – no rejection, no performance anxiety, and not having to worry about whether the person is enjoying it or not – what they ultimately equal is certainty. When we don't have to think about those three things, it gives us a high degree of certainty. In that moment of watching porn, certainty equals safety, and this is what we look for as human beings. Am I safe? Am I loved? These are the two needs that we're searching for all the time. So, when we're watching porn, we're highly safe. Everything's very safe, but it doesn't take us where we want to be going in the long term.

Conversations about porn seem like a taboo topic culturally and as a society. We don't talk about these kinds of things. We know it's there but it's this elephant in the room. But when it leads to not being able to get hard, not being able to have sex, and avoiding initiating intimacy because of awkwardness or embarrassment, the relationship's not going in a good direction. Even at that point, many couples still don't talk about it. They just avoid it or never talk about it, because it feels embarrassing or awkward.

* * *

We're all on the spectrum of addiction in some way, shape, or form, whether it is shopping, smartphones, porn, gambling, or food. When we think of addiction, we see addicts as people that society has cast away. We think of a drug addict injecting themselves on the street, but the reality is that we all have our addictions, although there are obviously levels of extremity. I think we all have a propensity for addiction because of the cycle that's created, whether it's social media or whether it's porn; it's quite easy to get into the cycle because of the needs that addiction meets.

Sometimes it is because of a relationship breakdown. We need to ask what part of ourselves we bring back home into the relationship. We can give everything to work, and we walk back through the door with whatever's left over and so that is not always a recipe for a 50/50 relationship. So, it becomes understandable why needs are not being met. Other things start to come into the picture. Porn being one of those things, infidelity being another, because someone else or something else is providing a higher form of stimulation.

* * *

Many of the men that I work with are either in senior positions in the workplace or have their own businesses, so they are experiencing a fairly high degree of pressure, whether it's pressure around finances and income, whether it's pressure to perform or perhaps, if they are younger, the pressure is coming from sport or maybe academics. I'm yet to find a guy where there have not been these external pressures, most of which started at a young age. It could be being compared to other children – 'Why can't you be like this other kid?' – or being ridiculed or shamed or guilted for not being good enough in the classroom.

So, these experiences start to sow the seeds of doubt about not being good enough. My performance in sport, or whatever it may be, is not good enough. And then we move into running our own businesses or having senior positions at work, and there's more pressure, higher expectations, higher stress. So, when one or two things don't go right, there's this pathway that is reignited in our minds that basically says, 'I'm not good enough.' It's performance anxiety, whether it's in the workplace, whether it's financial, whether it's in the bedroom – it is this pressure to perform, and the anxiety associated with 'What if I'm not good enough?' And so, outside of porn, these are the other things that play a role for many guys.

One example is a guy I've worked with, who for years and years had absolutely no challenges in the bedroom, with five kids, and had been married for 30 years. All of a sudden one night it just happened – he couldn't sustain an erection. And what was actually happening was that there were all these multiple other factors going on. There was a lot of pressure at work. He was thinking of buying his partner out of the business. The partner didn't really want to and that was a very difficult time. And there were also external pressures going on with his kids as well, and so often what we don't realise is that other contexts can impact our ability in the bedroom. What we can just lock into is, 'I haven't been able to get hard. What's wrong with me? I've got a problem.' And then we carry that thought through into the next time and starting thinking, 'I remember when this happened last time. It can't happen again. What if it happens again?' Pressure, pressure, pressure, and the thing that we don't want to happen happens – we lose the erection.

* * *

There can be a medical element to it, so the first thing to do is go and get a blood check and get a testosterone check as well. Most times – let's say with 80 per cent of the men I speak to – it's not medical; it's mindset. The easy thing to jump to, which we have to be aware of when we go and see a doctor, is pills – but that can then create a dependency cycle on the pills. Pills do not fix problems with mindset. They may give some short-term relief, but it certainly doesn't fix things in the long run.

The second thing is then try to take a step back and look at the context of the situation. Especially for men that perhaps feel like it just came out of nowhere, look at when it happened. Take a step back and think what else was going on in your life at that moment that could have – in some way, shape, or form – impacted what happened that night in the bedroom.

For men who have experienced this over a prolonged period, it may be going back to the first time they had sex, and it was not a good experience. Maybe things have happened on and off, but pretty much consistently over time. You do not have to accept that this is just how things are because you're 50 or 60 and it is just down to your age. It's comfortable to hide behind it being an age thing, but I've worked with guys from 17 up to 70, and it is not age, and you do not have to accept that this is just how life is going to be. It is about getting the right tools and strategies to get it sorted. And yes, it can feel awkward and uncomfortable to have that conversation with somebody, but my advice would be: what do you want for the rest of your life? You know, do you want it to just be this way? Potentially it will hold you back from being able to have a fulfilling connection, and passionate sex, which everybody deserves to experience. Do you want to not have those things so you can avoid having one or two awkward conversations that would help to get this sorted?

* * *

With performance anxiety comes a shitload of shame and doubt and self-guilt. All the time, 'I'm not good enough. What if I can't satisfy my partner? What if I'm not good enough for the person I want to attract into my life? Who am I? Am I even a real man if I can't do this?' We can question ourselves endlessly. Imagine that stacked over years and years and years. We basically hammer ourselves, you know, like the whack-a-mole game. I imagine it like that. We hammer ourselves down, down, and down into the ground until we're just this shell that just doesn't feel like ourselves any more, or we ask, 'Who am I in the world?' or 'What's my purpose in the world?' We become quite passive and draw back from relationships, avoid initiating intimacy, and avoid putting ourselves out there because we have all of these fears, all of this shame, all of this guilt. And that, stacked over years, is not going to lead anywhere good. And if you're in a relationship right now, there's only one direction it's going in – and it's not a good one.

It starts with us all as individuals and realising that we aren't going to suddenly wake up and find everything has been fixed for us, without us having to change anything, without experiencing a bit of 'ego discomfort.' It starts with us. By starting a conversation, whether it's with your partner, and saying, 'We both know this has been going on for a while and I don't have all the answers to it, but I know that I want to get this sorted and for us to build back the spark that we had in the bedroom.' Or whether it's reaching out to me, a different coach, a therapist, or your doctor. This is where it starts. And it's totally possible to feel normal again. You just have to take the first step, when you are ready to.

....

To contact Shay, visit his website at https://shay-doran.com or his YouTube channel at https://youtube.com/@shay-doran

CARL
FINDING YOUR CABIN
IN THE WOODS

'So, you carry on in life and something can trigger a memory. I can't say what because your mind will just go back and start popping open and, in my experience, when it pops open, you don't know what you're going to get.'

A few years back, I got diagnosed with quite severe PTSD. When the doctor did my tests, he didn't even bother to tell me how high it was. He said: 'We need to get you help, ASAP.' And it was virtually while we were having the conversation, he was making phone calls for me to see a counsellor.

Obviously, this upset me – his reaction to my diagnosis and how quickly he wanted me to be seen. It really rocked me on my feet. I had no idea that I was suffering from PTSD whatsoever. It was just a question of things that were happening at home. Bit of a short fuse on stupid little things. Major things didn't seem to bother me. For argument's sake, when somebody had washed up and put the cup standing up rather than turning it upside down – just crazy little things like that would rile me up.

I'd then think 'Why have I just done that?' and then just carry on. So, Sarah, my wife, sat me down and said, 'You're just not your normal self,' and we got talking and I just started bawling my eyes out. I'm not ashamed of it. She said, 'Right, we obviously need to get you down to the doctor's.' My dad came with me, and the doctor did a few tests and then hit me with the bombshell that there's a problem.

I then got an appointment with Oxfordshire Mental Health Plus, who were absolutely fantastic. The guy there was very chilled and when I wanted to do something or say something – it wasn't planned – he just said, 'We've got this time.' And then, after a few sessions, he said if it's okay with me, he'd like to start me off on a timeline. Can I remember events back in the past that might have upset me?

The earliest one I have is children playing in a park and there was one of those wooden banana boats that used to rock at a slight angle. They all jumped off of it for some reason or other, whatever they were playing, and I got hit on the forehead with it. Could that have been the start of something? I can't really tell.

We moved along the timeline. Anything else traumatic happened? There was the loss of my grandfather, who I was quite close to. I was about 14. It's quite dramatic losing a grandparent. That's what they call a Jack-in-the-Box. A memory, usually traumatic, that is tucked away in a box until it unexpectedly jumps out.

Then we move along to the next one – a car accident. Going through court, I found out that I wasn't actually speeding, but due to the weather conditions I put the brakes on too hard. There was a vehicle that had come off a building site, so my windscreen got covered with mud and rubbish. The wiper blades were going, I saw the brake lights go on, but due to my inexperience I swerved past it and then hit an oncoming vehicle. It's a hard-to-believe story, but it's a true story, that I actually hit a car that had four priests in it. So, it was either time to go or they were here to save me. I didn't realise it at the time until after the impact when I was laid out of the car on the road. I think the adrenaline really kicked in and my heartbeat must have gone way out of its normal zone, when I saw one of the priests coming over to me with his hands looming down towards my head, and I was just gone – I went unconscious.

The next thing I know, I'm in the back of the ambulance. Looking back, it was quite surreal, but at the time I remember waking up and looking around and thinking, 'Where did the priest go?' and one of the paramedics looked at me and said: 'Oh, he's back with us.' I remember him shouting to his colleague 'Everything's okay' and then I was unconscious again.

I woke up in the hospital a couple of hours later or so, towards the evening, and the two paramedics actually came and saw me. 'It's unbelievable,' they told me. I had hit a group of priests in their car. Oh my God! I started to have a bit of recall, but nothing more after seeing the priest come down towards my head and then waking up in the ambulance. They said: 'We've been to a lot of RTAs [road traffic accidents] and we recommend that you keep wearing your St Christopher because normally, nine times out of ten, you would have been in a bag, and we'd have been doing some paperwork.' So, there's another Jack-in-the-Box.

I remember I was just lying in hospital thinking, 'Why do I hurt so much?' But the pain eventually went, and I was out of hospital, and I carried on with life and I just looked back and thought, 'Well, that was a funny moment.' I survived it and I thought, 'Well, it's not my time to go.'

Then I had a big incident at work. I'm a security officer. I was one of the nominated first-aiders but I was newly qualified – less than a week – and was called to an incident and had to give CPR to somebody and I just did what I had to do. We then had a first responder turn up who just happened to work on our site and was going home but had his kit with him, and we were all just trying to save this person. We had two paramedics turn up and we explained the situation to them and that we'd done CPR several times and that we had got him back, he was breathing, and then he had gone again. It had happened a couple of times where he had sat up, spoken to us, and then he'd just be gone again. We found out later from his employer that he had a heart condition.

At the same time, my wife was in the ward above at the same hospital suffering from a blockage to the lungs and heart following an operation. So, knowing she was in there too was on my mind as I was trying to deal with the patient.

When we had to get the ambulance out to my wife and we got to A&E, the doctor said to me, 'Give it another half hour and you'd have been signing some different paperwork.' And that is another Jack-in-the-Box.

So, you carry on in life and something can trigger a memory. I can't say what because your mind will just go back and start popping open and, in my experience, when it pops open, you don't know what you're going to get.

Sometime after, I had a bit of a relapse and had to have several months off work, well, half a year – and then, a couple of months back, I had another bit of a relapse. Sometimes you can feel those triggers coming and sometimes they just hit you. But hopefully, when you get hit by that trigger, you have some way of getting some help. That's the biggest thing I can say to anybody. I can't really tell you what you've got to do; but in my experience, get help.

It sometimes needs to be that person in front of you who's trained and who can understand what you're going through. It's not necessarily something in the here and now that's triggered you – it could be something in the past and that's what we refer to as Jack-in-the-Boxes. When they pop open, it's not slow, you don't have time to push them back down, but you need to be aware and try and stop them before you get to that trigger point rather than leaving it too late, because you really don't want to have to go through it again.

You've got to try and be strong in yourself and let other people help you, but you've also got to do it yourself. It's only you who knows what's going on in your mind and how you feel. You can say something, but are you actually feeling it? It's a lot like fight or flight. You can choose flight and blag it, but actually the person in front of you is trying to help, so you have to give the absolute truth, no matter how much it hurts.

* * *

So, when I was told it was PTSD, I thought: 'I now know what it is, but can you tell me about it and what can I do?' By chance, my wife was just scrolling through Facebook and said to me: 'You like going out on your bike and for a walk, but you're always alone. South Moreton Boxing Club is doing a thing with men's mental health, chats, and helping you in the gym.' So, I got in contact with Steve, a great bloke who is nice and friendly to approach and who you can easily talk to. The club has now become my cabin in the woods.

Everybody needs a cabin in the woods, whether it's a hobby or just time for yourself. It's not a selfish thing. It's just great to have an environment where I can get myself fitter and stronger because you think: 'Oh God, I can't live this way.' Well, you can't live that way, so in the gym you might say to yourself you can lift seven kilograms. Well, that's your first positive step. And then you try another seven and suddenly you're lifting

14 kilograms. You've got to see that as a positive. So, you are getting physically stronger but you're also achieving something. It's a challenge, but it's an achievable challenge.

At the club, it's just nice that I can have that little bit of 'me' time – my cabin in the woods. If I want to talk, I can do, or I can choose to hit the bag a little bit harder just to get rid of the stress. It's controlled and I don't end up in any trouble. It's somewhere I look forward to going to. I work shifts, so I don't come here at regular times so it's different every day – so I might see different people and it's always nice to see Steve because we have a little chat, although for some reason we always end up on food, which isn't helpful when you're in the gym.

The more people that are diagnosed with mental health and are brave enough to talk to other people about it, the better. I think that's one of the real problems with mental health; it doesn't matter whether it's PTSD, anxiety, or depression, the first thing to do is to have contact with either a professional or hopefully they've got an understanding family. Luckily, my family, my dad and my wife, told me I wasn't my normal self, and I think we all know why now.

My advice to anyone feeling like I did – for example, frustrated by small things – is to try and take a step back from the situation. Don't let it get out of hand. You kind of have to go through hell a little bit with yourself. I don't mean in a nasty way, but it's kind of like self-healing but you've got other people there to help you.

Provided other people realise that sometimes you need that little check: 'Everything okay? How's your day?', 'Yes, okay. No problems really.' You know, you just need a conversation with somebody, either a professional or very good friends, to have a little chat, you know, and just to be okay.

There are warning signs once you've been diagnosed, and hopefully you'll know how to spot them. I wouldn't say it's like walking through a minefield for the rest of your life, because you then start worrying about stuff. You just carry on as normal as possible. Then just realise if something goes wrong – for example, you spill some milk or something like that – just don't make a big thing about it. It's an accident. Whose fault was it, really? It was nobody else's other than your own. You know, I'm not saying that your mental illness that you've been diagnosed with is your fault; there are obviously circumstances that have put you there, but just be aware of how you got there. I think that's the most important thing to be aware of – how you got there.

It's like I say to Steve [at the boxing club], if you are a broken crayon, you can still colour, and there's a message within that, which is that the word 'broken' contains the letters 'O' and 'K'.

The more people who suffer from PTSD and are dealing with it and can talk about it with other people out there, hopefully the more people are mindful. We can't always have it in the front of our mind, but try and be considerate – try to be kind to other people. I think there's kindness in all of us. There's hopefulness in all of us. It's whether we choose to open that door, and thankfully I've got a lot of people willing to do that. When you walk through that door, if you're going to be scared, it's better to be scared of something you know.

ANDREA
MENOPAUSE MADE SIMPLE: WHAT MEN SHOULD KNOW

'Say things like, "I'm worried about you." Or "What I've noticed is…" That is the easiest way to open up a conversation or to pick up on someone telling you that perhaps they're struggling … Please do not ask that question at three in the morning when you're both tetchy from lack of sleep, and she's sweating like a marathon runner in the desert wearing a fleece. Now is not a good time for that conversation.'

It's really my experience that makes me want to engage as many men as possible in this conversation. We often think of menopause as simply just a time in life when periods stop and women might have a few hot flushes and night sweats. My experience and the experience of many other women was more about the negative impact that menopause had on my mental health. This is especially why men need to know because, as a woman, if your mental health isn't in a good place and you're in a relationship, be it marriage or partnership, or just in the work environment, it's just worth as many men as possible knowing that there is a lot more to it than hot flushes and night sweats.

There is also the humour or banter around menopause – you know, a woman in a T-shirt in the middle of winter, standing by an open window with a fan in her hand; it's how we tend to think of it – but there is actually a very serious side too. From my own experience, my mental health was so badly affected that I made a plan to end my life.

What I now know is that I am not alone, and many other women will go through challenges of that nature. In fact, it is said that as many as 10 per cent of perimenopausal women will have thoughts of suicide due to the rollercoaster of hormones that's happening around that time, and there are lots of statistics that show that the issue is much, much wider and much, much bigger than perhaps the humour might suggest.

I'm a woman on a mission to get as many people informed and aware as possible. It's not only about looking after the female in your life but, from a man's perspective, it's also about recognising the impact it can have on relationships, the impact that it can have on sexual intimacy, the impact that it can have in terms of the divorce rates.

What we need to start recognising is that it's a perfectly normal, natural human transition and it is something that will affect 51 per cent of the population directly, but – the chances are – 100 per cent of the population indirectly.

So, for a man, I think it's worth understanding just the basic information about menopause. You certainly don't need to be an expert. You don't need to be able to score ten out of ten in a pub quiz, but it's just about realising the basic stuff, such as, in the UK, the average age for menopause for a white female is 51. That number is simply the date that signifies 12 months previously without any menstrual bleeding. However, the bit that we often overlook is that until we get to that point, the hormones are on a massive rollercoaster ride for on average four years prior to menopause, and in some cases it can be as long as 12 years.

During that time, what's happening is hormone levels are fluctuating up and down, and it's the fluctuation that causes the issue. What men may notice is perhaps a change in mood or a change in energy levels. It might be that your team member, your partner, or your wife is a little bit more tetchy than usual, perhaps a little bit forgetful. And again, we joke about things like brain fog, but if you're, for example, a woman in the workplace and you're experiencing that brain fog where you just can't find the words that you're looking for, not only can that be embarrassing, but that can also be career-ending. Many women actually consider whether to give up work because of the cognitive effect of those perimenopausal symptoms.

There are 34 symptoms of menopause, basically head to toe, and it affects all our major systems. It can affect brain health, cardiac health, and digestive health. It certainly has an impact on the major organs – the liver, the kidneys, the heart, etc. – because the key thing that's happening is hormone levels are rising and falling and eventually petering out. Hormones are not just required for sexual reproduction. Hormones are required for the brain, the heart, and the stomach. We have more than 300 bodily functions that are reliant on that steady source of hormones and it doesn't take a genius to work out that if those levels start to fluctuate and all those different body systems are not getting the hormones they need, then absolutely you experience changes in mood and behaviour, insomnia, vasomotor problems, the whole thing with temperatures and sweating and flushes. Heart palpitations are another common symptom, because the heart needs a supply of oestrogen, which is fluctuating.

What I'd like men to realise is that there's a lot more to this than they perhaps immediately appreciate and that it can affect everything from thinning hair at the top of your head to aching joints around your feet. Every single bodily function is affected by those hormones.

* * *

In terms of what men need to say – and this is perhaps a little bit tongue-in-cheek, and why I've named my latest book *Could It Be Your Hormones, Love?* – there is definitely a question that I want men to be comfortable asking. However, ask it at the right time with the right tone of voice and in the right context so that you don't risk getting your head ripped off.

So, 'Could it be your hormones, love?' and all the questions that you might want to ask a menopausal woman are really there to just start the conversation, but make sure you start it from a place of concern, not from a place of judgement or criticism.

Say things like, 'I'm worried about you.' Or 'What I've noticed is…' That is the easiest way to open up a conversation or to pick up on someone telling you that perhaps they're struggling, you know, 'I'm really struggling. I don't know what's wrong with me.' And you reply, 'Okay. Talk to me about it. Have you spoken to anybody else about this?' And that is a perfect 'Could it be your hormones, love?' conversation as long as that question is asked in the right tone of voice with very positive intent. Please do not ask that question at three in the morning when you're both tetchy from lack of sleep, and she's sweating like a marathon runner in the desert wearing a fleece. Now is not a good time for that conversation. So, choose your moment at a time when you can both have a grown-up conversation about something that perhaps might feel a little bit uncomfortable.

One of the biggest challenges is lack of knowledge. I think as recently as 2021, research was done where more than 80 per cent of women said they had very little or no knowledge and understanding of perimenopause. And if you think about it, perimenopause is quite a new word in our vocabulary. We've only just got used to talking about menopause and now we want to talk about perimenopause. *Peri* is the Greek word for 'about' or 'around', so basically it's the time around that menopause date.

When we're at school, we get lessons in biology, about puberty and periods and how to not get pregnant – hopefully

– and then, when we leave school, if we do get pregnant there's a whole plethora of information out there. There are books, magazines, and all sorts of stuff where women can access knowledge and information about things like the size of your embryo today and what's happening to it. But once you get past those procreative years, nobody comes along and says, 'Oh, excuse me, let me tell you about the menopause 'cause that's coming next and you need to be aware.' There's a campaign going to Parliament at the moment that's asking for women to start to receive education and medical appointments once they reach the age of 40 to 45.

We have seen some tragic circumstances where women have been misdiagnosed because the other missing piece in the jigsaw is that general practitioner doctors are not routinely trained in menopause. As many as 40 per cent of UK universities don't even have menopause on the syllabus for medical graduates. It's only from 2024 that it will be something that is routinely covered.

I'm not here to bash GPs, because if nobody's taught them, how are they supposed to know? But it seems a bit silly that a condition that affects 51 per cent of the population isn't a routine area of study, especially as we now know that it can lead to suicide. It's definitely something we need to be paying more attention to.

So, women don't know, GPs don't know, so somebody needs to. Maybe this is where we turn to the men in our lives and say, 'Come on! Be the cheerleader, be the expert, step up!'

★ ★ ★

There is no such thing as a typical menopause. Every woman is different. The lead-up is on average four years but in some cases 10 to 12 years. Then once the day of the menopause arrives, i.e. 12 months without any menstrual bleed, we are then postmenopausal, and nothing changes from then on in. We don't suddenly find a cache of hormones that were previously hidden. We are now without those hormones, and that is then lifelong. What we know tends to happen is the symptoms tend to sort of peter out over time but can last for as much as six years post-menopause. That's why more and more medical professionals are now pushing for hormone replacement therapy, because we now know that HRT can have positive health benefits, not just around menopause, but also when it comes to conditions like osteoporosis, cardiovascular disease, and dementia. For example, twice as many women are diagnosed with dementia and there's some great research looking at whether it could be to do with those hormones that peter out during menopause.

So, we've been looking at what you might call *natural* menopause, but we do also need to be mindful that some women can have what we might call a *medical* or *surgical* menopause. For example, if a woman has to have a hysterectomy or ovaries removed or indeed undergoes any treatment such as chemotherapy, it can bring on menopause sooner. It really is something that's a much bigger subject than we necessarily first thought.

Even though the average age for a Caucasian woman to go through menopause in the UK is 51, one in a hundred women will go through menopause in their forties. One in a thousand will go through it even earlier than that. We rely on the biological system that we have from birth and there are circumstances where menopause can happen at a much younger age, or overnight, so you don't have that rollercoaster, that lead-up to it, that you would have if it was a natural menopause.

* * *

It's not just the physiological signs and symptoms; there are also the psychological ones. This is the area I am particularly passionate about given my own lived experience and also the professional work that I've been doing for many years.

One thing that we need to understand is the brain has oestrogen receptors. Now, those receptors are not there for ornament or decoration – the brain needs oestrogen to function well. It also needs progesterone, which is important to the calming of our parasympathetic system, so our nervous system.

For example, if a woman experiences stress, as with a man, cortisol and adrenaline are released and that's what creates anxiety. It's the hormone progesterone that will typically calm that impact and therefore help us to then relax and de-stress. If progesterone is one of those hormones that's in decline during perimenopause, immediately you start to appreciate the stress effect for a menopausal woman because the hormone isn't there to calm it, so I believe that menopause starts in the brain. Through the reading and the research that I've done, we will tend to experience symptoms at head level far sooner. And that can be anything from that brain fog where you can't quite find the words. It might be memory. You might struggle to retain information. So again, using the example of a woman in the workplace, perhaps being introduced to a new software system, and she is suddenly finding herself having to ask the same question over and over. It's not that she's stupid. It's simply that the ability to retain information is being negatively affected in the brain.

Other issues at a head level – and again this one is often the subject of banter – is when you can't quite find the right word. For some reason during menopause, nouns go missing completely and you just don't know what that thing is called any more – and that can be quite funny if you look at it one way. But if you actually understand and appreciate what's going on at a far deeper level, then the brain isn't quite firing on all cylinders because it's not being nourished and fed by the hormones it needs.

The other issue is the impact on levels of serotonin, which affects mood, especially positive mood. If those serotonin levels are affected, as they can be, then we can experience low mood or depression. An increasing number of women are reporting anxiety who've never experienced anxiety at any point in their lives previously. And that anxiety can then have some quite significant knock-on effects.

I'm aware of women who've left work. I'm aware of women who've stopped driving because they're too anxious to simply get behind the wheel of a car. And those kinds of behaviours, as I'm sure you'll appreciate, can significantly impact not only that person's lifestyle and way of being but can also start to impact on things like self-esteem. That then creates tension in relationships, because if you're my husband and you've no clue what's going on, and all of a sudden I don't want to drive, or I don't think I'm capable of doing my job, or I worry about where the children are and why aren't they home, because typically they're teenagers by this point or slightly older. So, you can see why it can cause a lot of tension in relationships, as well as a massive impact on a person's self-esteem, self-belief, self-confidence, and self-worth.

Then if we also consider that, at that time in life, perhaps children are going off to university and you've got a whole change of life, so that can bring on empty nest syndrome. Women who are perhaps in their late forties, or early fifties, at the pinnacle of their career, perhaps they're responsible for a team, perhaps they're responsible for a whole department – the stress that goes with that. And let's not forget that lovely phrase, the 'sandwich generation', whereby we're at an age now where we're looking after older children, but we also find ourselves caring for elderly relatives. So, being in that sandwich generation can be really stressful, and absolutely a lot of men will have those same challenges, but statistically it still falls to the woman of the house to take care of those responsibilities, those caring duties. Many women have got stuff going on internally with that hormone imbalance, but are also often leading busy, stressful lives where their own self-care is a long way down the list of priorities.

That is often why we don't notice, because women say things like, 'Oh, I'm just a bit busy at the minute; there's nothing wrong with me.' Or 'What do you mean I'm forgetful? Well, I'm bound to be, aren't I? You know, I'm juggling all of these things.' I was even in a situation where my period stopped and they put that down to the stress that I was undergoing at that time, when in hindsight I was perimenopausal and needed some help.

* * *

The risk of suicidal thoughts increases by a factor of seven during this time, and if you look at the Office for National Statistics numbers you'll see that the most substantial number of female deaths by suicide is between the ages of 45 and 49. I don't think that's a coincidence. I think there's just so much going on internally and externally that leaves a woman potentially feeling hopeless and worthless. This is the part that men can play, to encourage us to ask for the help we need, to challenge perhaps when the GP says, 'Oh, you're not old enough for menopause,' but actually they've never studied it. They've got no idea about it and women will need to advocate for themselves. There is definitely a key part for men to play during this time – helping to look out for signs, helping to provide support, and making sure that the load is spread.

It is suggested that during this time – say, between the ages of 40 and 59 – divorce rates increase significantly, and recent research by a law firm tells us that 62 per cent of divorces are instigated by menopausal women. I think this is down to a combination of factors: there are the debilitating effects that menopause symptoms can have, and there's also an increased risk of tension and stress in relationships because things like sexual intimacy can be affected. The impact of the lack of hormones can affect a woman's libido but also create vaginal dryness, a condition that means that intercourse can be excruciatingly painful. Bedroom intimacy can cause issues in relationships, and I've certainly heard of many cases where people have been accused of having affairs because they haven't wanted to engage in intimacy, but it is actually down to a hormonal imbalance.

We also know though, let's be honest, maybe it's a bit of a *Thelma and Louise* moment. Maybe women get to the point where they think, 'You know what, this is my second spring' – which is what Chinese medicine refers to menopause as – 'and I don't want to spend it in a situation where I'm just not living to my full potential. Maybe I am just going to walk out the door.' I know plenty of women for whom an apartment overlooking the sea – with solo occupancy that doesn't take children or pets – has become a bit of a dream. So be aware; be very aware.

My best piece of advice is to get comfortable with the uncomfortable. Start to learn, understand, and become more aware. If you're in a workplace where they are sensibly offering menopause awareness or they've got a menopause-friendly policy, get involved and understand it. If you are a husband or partner of someone and you wonder whether it's happening to them, do your homework, do some research, and create an opportunity to have a really useful conversation. I fundamentally believe that conversations can change relationships. Conversations can save lives. So, get comfortable with the uncomfortable and get talking about it.

....

Andrea is the author of *Could It Be Your Hormones, Love?* and her website is https://inherrightmind.com/.

SHAWN

PSYCHEDELICS, NATURE, AND HEALING AFTER CORPORATE LIFE

'The mind is really, really adept at insulating us from really, really difficult or traumatic experiences. Think about people who have endured really significant abuse at some point in their life or in early childhood. It's not uncommon for individuals to have no conscious recollection of those memories … The psychedelic experience often provides a window to begin to explore the parts of ourselves that are suppressed, the parts of ourselves where we may have difficulties.'

I've recently begun a second career. I spent 25 years in corporate America working primarily in supply chain. Just a few years ago, my role with a large retailer was eliminated out of the blue. Even when I was receiving the news, I knew I was receiving a gift – I just didn't at that time quite understand the nature of that gift.

Approximately 15 years ago, I started addressing my challenges with depression and anxiety by seeing a therapist and by seeking medication. I joke that my relationship with my personal therapist is almost longer than with anyone in my life beyond my nuclear family. I've been seeing the same therapist since 2009, and I see him every week. I can't quite imagine not having that support in my life, both for me personally and to aid me in my current work as a psychotherapist.

In 2021, I started a master's in a social work programme, with the intent of becoming a therapist myself. I finished that degree a little over a year ago, and I currently practise under what's called supervision at a small private practice in the Twin Cities of Minnesota.

I've been married, divorced, and since remarried, but my first marriage I often describe as a mirror that I was not prepared to see my reflection in, and that relationship prompted me to begin to understand, initially just on the surface, just how much I was struggling with my own mental health. She and I had started marital counselling and that made it clear to me that seeking some individual support would likely be helpful. Little did I know how helpful it would be.

But it was clear – even ten years ago, maybe even longer – that there were whispers of 'Hmm, you know, there are parts of your job that you really don't enjoy.' And those whispers began in my mind, but I had already kind of made up a narrative that the hurdles were too high, like going back to school for two years, and working under supervised practice, wasn't reasonable. And then of course, income – I'm not going to make as much money as a therapist as I was working as a leader in corporate America. But those whispers were present, and I think they eventually became shouts, and the universe works in mysterious and beautiful ways. Losing my job was just a shove. It was just a kick in the ass that, in retrospect, I really needed and I'm grateful for it. As I mentioned, there was a part of me that was grateful for it even as I was getting the news, because I knew there was something good on the other side of whatever this hurdle was or was not.

Then I rested. I very much rested. And hindsight provides so much clarity but, on some level, I rested for almost two years. And during that time, I got to be a dad, a stepdad, a husband, a friend, a son, and a brother.

In early 2020, and by this point I'd read Michael Pollan's book *How to Change Your Mind*, I had a really strong interest in psychedelics and how it may aid people who struggle with various aspects of their mental health. In college, in my early years, I'd had some experience with psychedelics in kind of a party setting would be the best way to describe it, but eventually I chose to attend a psilocybin mushroom retreat in Jamaica. I'm a deeply intuitive person and I just felt, in my gut, that this would be a really good thing to do.

Probably my greatest hurdle was trying to explain to my wife what I wanted to do and why I wanted to do it, because her initial response was, 'You want to do what and where, and it's going to cost what?' But she eventually warmed to the idea.

There were 11 of us, all from the US, that travelled down there for this retreat, and it was led by four US-based therapists. Their approach was quite similar to that taken at Johns Hopkins University in terms of some of the clinical studies that have been done, so there is a bit of a ceremonial feel to the environment. As part of the experience, you're typically wearing an eye mask to block out that part of your senses, and you're either listening to a curated playlist or wearing headphones and listening to music. You're lying on a mat. The music and the mask are really kind of forcing you a bit inward into your experience of the medicine.

And I refer to these things, whether it's psilocybin or some of the other psychedelics, like they are truly medicine – medicines that have been used in some cases for thousands of years. I think we're still uncovering and understanding the history of some of these compounds and how they've aided humanity in various ways for a very long time.

And you're guided, which is incredibly important. If you were to tackle one of these things on your own, it's not a good idea, so having a skilled facilitator is really important.

It might mean that just that guide, that therapist, is simply present. They're just there should you need support or encounter some distress that you're not able to move through on your own. But it's somebody that's just present for you and has a really deep understanding of what you're going through and what you might experience.

And it kind of prompts the question of what are you going through? There's a famous neuroscientist by the name of Sam Harris, and one of the things that he articulates is that there's a poverty of words and language to describe what these experiences are. Broadly, psychedelics propel you into a non-ordinary state of consciousness. So, it can be a very, very intense experience that can be confusing. There could be both auditory and visual hallucinations, but you're entering a part of your unconscious mind in a way that no other kind of ordinary state of consciousness is really similar to.

The mind is really, really adept at insulating us from really, really difficult or traumatic experiences. Think about people who have endured really significant abuse at some point in their life or in early childhood. It's not uncommon for individuals to have no conscious recollection of those memories. Fortunately, that wasn't my experience early in life, but the psychedelic experience often provides a window to begin to explore the parts of ourselves that are suppressed, the parts of ourselves where we may have difficulties.

The truth of the matter is that we don't fully understand how these things work, but one of the things that Michael Pollan references in his book is the concept of neuroplasticity, which is essentially just the degree to which habits or patterns are embedded in our brain and cause us to get stuck in certain ways – and probably addiction is the best example of this. In a way, we develop ruts in our brain that are ways of behaviour that are really difficult to overcome. He describes how an intense psychedelic experience can be like a fresh coat of snow over a mountain that covers up the ruts and provides the opportunity to develop new neural pathways, which enable us to tackle aspects of our behaviour that have negatively impacted our mental health.

What we think happens is that psychedelics can accelerate neural growth and create opportunities for neurogenesis for actual physical changes in our brain. But, like I said, these are somewhat poorly understood. Yet we know that, in some of the trials, people will report that a psychedelic experience is in the top five spiritual experiences of their life. So, it's a really powerful modality that is still kind of gaining traction and acceptance in the world.

I think about being a child in the 1980s and the narrative around the effects on the brain from these types of drugs – that mushrooms are drugs, and these things are really toxic and to be avoided at all costs. So, there are significant cultural headwinds, probably not just in the US but throughout the world, that these compounds had no redeeming medical or societal value.

* * *

I've struggled with anxiety my whole life and I returned from Jamaica as the pandemic was hitting in March of 2020. There was a lot of fear in the world. My kids were obviously much younger then, and we were migrating to remote learning. There was a lot of chaos in the world, and I had never felt so calm and grounded in my life.

During that retreat, it was very clear that the path for me was to pursue a new career in mental health. It still took me several months to apply to schools and eventually enrol in a programme and begin the process, but it was pretty rapid after I returned and, ultimately, I started my master's programme in the fall of 2021, the following year. I had rested for two years, and it took me a while to even acknowledge how much my career had taken out of me and recognise that I needed the time of rest and reflection and anchoring back to the things that were most important in my life.

I think a part of my journey was just learning to love and accept myself. The culture in corporate life and just in culture more broadly of 'never being good enough' is so prolific. I mean, in truth, I think a big part of our economies depend on people having an orientation to themselves of never being good enough. In my roles and corporate life, the expectations of 'Oh, well, this is what you achieved this quarter, but you gotta do better next quarter, next year.' Never being good enough was always a theme with my responsibilities and the teams that I led, but I attached really readily to just this deep-seated fear in me that I wasn't good enough. And so, I had participated in that model for so long, in a way that became a part of my identity – of not being good enough.

So, for me, almost by definition, it really didn't permit me to come forward, because I was operating from a place of fear that these deeply held views were true. My outside environment really validated my insecurities and my inability to love and accept myself. And this might be a little bit over the top but, in a way, the environments that I worked in exploited something that already existed within me.

★ ★ ★

Halfway through my master's programme I had kind of a serendipitous opportunity to travel deep into the jungles of Peru for two weeks on an ayahuasca retreat. It was interesting because I was familiar with ayahuasca – it's arguably one of the most powerful psychedelic substances on the planet – but it wasn't really high on my list of priorities. However, I was introduced via an acquaintance in my hometown to an individual who had a passion for psychedelics as it applies to the world of mental health, and it became really clear that this was something to explore.

During just short of two weeks in the jungle of Peru, I attended a retreat called Casa del Maestro and met Maestro Alberto, who is the *ayahuasquero*, the shaman who led this retreat. This is an individual who had worked in this capacity in his community, in his culture, since he was a very young boy.

I participated in five ceremonies over the course of six days. The ceremonies happened in the evening, beginning at eight o'clock, and took place in a circular building called the *maloca*, utilised for this purpose. The ayahuasca ceremony itself is a kind of tea and you ingest a relatively small amount of it. It doesn't taste particularly good – and the amount that you drink, you decide on your own and in concert with the shaman. Maestro would lead the ceremony along with one or more of his sons and a couple of other facilitators. In this case, one was an American from upstate New York, and another a Russian, originally from Siberia, to put the ceremony into Western language.

The interesting part about ayahuasca is that the shaman and other facilitators are ingesting the medicine with you. It can last anywhere from two to five hours, and the experience, or at least my experience, was that the shaman led the intensity of the experience and played a role in what takes place in the ceremony. I explored that with them afterwards and they told me they're in contact with the spirits that are present among us.

Some people are sitting in chairs around the circumference of the maloca, while others might be lying on mattresses in the middle. It's an intense inward journey. It's dark. You're not wearing a mask, but it's dark. You can't see a whole lot. And one of the things that struck me is just the profound stillness of the experience. Maestro Alberto and those leading it are singing songs that they call *icaros*, which are specific songs that they sing in the ceremony, and at times they would break from singing and just be silent for a bit.

And then you would just hear the sounds of the jungle. And it felt like everything in the jungle was in the maloca with you and that everything was working in concert with one another to make the experience what it was. And if I think about what I avoided so much in my life prior to starting this journey, it was just stillness and being with myself and being alone with my thoughts.

Sometimes my thoughts were dark, intrusive, and scary. But everything's working together and everything's as it is. And we try and accept what's taking place at that moment without judgement, without trying to change it, without all the sideways thoughts that kind of get in our way and prompt anxiety and fear and distress.

I would say the most profound experience I had was my fourth night in the maloca. My dad passed away in January of

2015 and I always knew that he had suffered from something that he never described to me during his time on earth. That fourth night, I spent with him. In a way, I relived some of the traumatic experiences that he experienced. Honestly, it was the most challenging experience of my life. I was begging God to end it because of how afraid I was. In the middle of the experience, I didn't know what it was about, and towards the end I realised what it was and who it was about, and it was about my dad. I felt his physical presence that night in a way that was not unlike when he was alive and when he hugged me and told me that he was proud of me.

And this experience fundamentally changed me as a human being. I know that my dad is present with me every day in the work that I do, in my life, and in my relationships. And yeah, it changed me – and, in a way, it didn't change me. It just connected me to my own authenticity and who I am.

In many respects, it just furthered what was already in place in terms of my perception of how these substances can help us. It really kind of cracked my heart open and anchored me to a sense of interconnectedness and spirituality that I didn't have before. And I think that's a common thread in all psychedelics, but one that was most profound for me when I was in Peru is that as people, as human beings, we're all deeply interconnected in ways that are both really clear and really subtle.

And then it also connected me to nature and all things in our environment, whether that's living things like trees, rocks, or just everything that makes up the earth. I've always been kind of connected to trees, and part of the traditions of the Peruvian people and this medicine is that all the trees, all the plants, have spirits – and spirits that are able to help us and to provide clarity on how we're connected to them and one another. So, the ayahuasca intensified my connection with nature. I like to go into Northern Minnesota, into the wilderness by myself, for short periods of time, just to go be with the trees.

Today we have all these pharmaceutical approaches to mental health but we're so far away from nature. I have this theory that maybe a thousand years ago a medicine person and a culture might have prescribed going to the woods for two weeks by yourself and come back and you will be healed.

The windows in my office face trees and then beyond the trees is a pond and some water. And I know that in a way these trees outside my office help me; they help the work that's going on in my office. And it's funny, as I say these things, if the me of three or four years ago heard me speak, I would say I'm nuts. You know, I'm kind of off. I'm way out in left field. And yet it's a function of what I've learned. So, with some of my clients will I reference how I believe the trees are helping us in that room? Absolutely. And encouraging individuals to go for a walk in nature – it's something that I suggest all the time.

With my colleagues, we often joke or speculate that, if all of our clients went for a 30-minute walk outside every day, our business would collapse, although that's probably a bit of an exaggeration.

I don't want to oversimplify the challenges that people face. You know, movement and nature, I think they're part of what can just naturally connect us back to ourselves. That's always been true, and I don't believe it will ever not be true.

Something that I think underpins all of it is mycelium, which is the precursor to the fruits that eventually become fungi and mushrooms and essentially cover the earth; they are kind of the original internet. They are the pathways by which nature might communicate to redirect resources to a plant or a tree that might be struggling. We're learning that plant life is intelligent, and I think that's part of how a connection with nature helps us heal. Going out and walking on the earth without shoes, and just putting your feet in the earth, I think is something that can be really grounding and really powerful. In fact, as I prepare for sessions with clients, sometimes I will visualise anchoring myself back to the earth, back to the very core of the earth, visualise my feet walking in the grass, walking in the woods, just to ground myself so I'm better equipped to support those that I'm working with.

I think there is an intelligence and the more open we are to it, the more access we have to the power that this is. I think our systems are such that these concepts seem a little woo-woo or out there. They also aren't a source of revenue and the 'never being good enough' piece is so hyper-connected to money, to resources and separating us from connecting back to ourselves and the world that surrounds us.

I think about it as like there's a cost to everything and we've got all these technological advances and these phones that we're all connected to, and there's a lot of really positive parts to these innovations, but there's also a cost. I think we're developing a different awareness of what the costs are of not being in connection and relationship with people, spending time in person with people versus connecting on social media or via text or things of that nature. There are a lot of people who don't even want a phone call any more – and not only do we need phone calls, but we need physical contact. We need to hug. We need to see the whites of one another's eyes and be in connection and a community with others. I think overarching to all this is that we heal in relationships. We don't heal in isolation. It's not possible.

My advice is to be vulnerable. How do you identify what it is that's causing you distress and how do you find someone that you trust to be vulnerable with? I'm a therapist, but there are so many experiences in life that are therapy, like going and having coffee with a friend. Having somebody to talk to about things like 'I've really been struggling with my relationship with my partner, with my children, with myself' – that's therapy. Going and walking in the woods is therapy. I would say find a way to identify what's happening and take that first step to be vulnerable with another human being who you trust – and that doesn't have to be a therapist. There are no requirements other than find someone that you trust. Because I think, particularly for men, there are hurdles about what is therapy and what does that mean about me as a man, as a human being? It's not a sign of weakness; it's a sign of strength.